MOCKTAIL
SYRUPS & CORDIALS

EASILY ELEVATE YOUR NON-ALCOHOLIC DRINK CREATIONS

BOOK 3 of the *Mocktails for Every Day* series

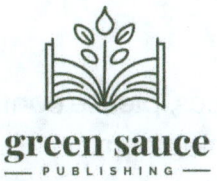

green sauce
PUBLISHING

Copyright Notice
© 2025 Green Sauce. All rights reserved.

No part of this book may be reproduced, stored in a retrieval system, or transmitted in any form or by any means—electronic, mechanical, photocopying, recording, or otherwise—without the prior written permission of the publisher, except in the case of brief quotations used in reviews or critical articles.

The publisher is not responsible for any adverse effects resulting from the use of the recipes, ingredients or information provided in this book.

For permissions or inquiries, please contact:
info@greensaucepublishing.com

TABLE OF CONTENTS

INTRODUCTION 1

SIMPLE SYRUPS

Basil Syrup 15
Berry Syrup 16
Chili-Infused Syrup 17
Caramel Syrup 18
Coconut Syrup 19
Cinnamon Syrup 20
Chocolate Syrup 21
Dill Syrup 22
Ginger Syrup 23
Grenadine Syrup 24
Honey Syrup 25
Hibiscus Syrup 26
Lavender Syrup 27
Jasmine Syrup 28
Lemongrass Syrup 29
Lemon Syrup 30
Lime Syrup 31
Maple Pecan Syrup 32
Orange Zest Syrup 33
Mint Syrup 34
Orange Syrup 35
Peach Syrup 36
Pumpkin Spice Syrup 37
Peppermint Syrup 38
Rose Syrup 39
Raspberry Syrup 40
Spiced Clove Syrup 41
Rosemary Syrup 42
Tamarind Syrup 43
Vanilla Bean Syrup 44

TABLE OF CONTENTS

Violet Syrup **45**
Thyme Syrup **46**
Spiced Syrup **47**
Honey-Ginger Syrup **48**

INFUSIONS
Cinnamon **53**
Clove and Orange **54**
Mint Infusion **55**
Hibiscus Tea **56**
Mulling Spice **57**
Herb-Infused Water **58**
Pumpkin Spice Glow **59**
Chai Concentrate **60**
Citrus Infusion **61**

CORDIALS
Elderflower Cordial **65**
Lemon Cordial **66**
Spiced Apple Cordial **67**
Lime Cordial **68**
Rosemary Cordial **69**

NUT MILKS
Macadamia Nut Milk **74**
Classic Almond Nut Milk **75**
Brazil Nut Milk **76**
Toasted Hazelnut Milk **77**
Pecan Nut Milk **78**
Walnut Milk **79**

The Secret to Extraordinary Mocktails!

What's the secret to a truly amazing mocktail? It's not just the fresh fruit, the perfect balance of flavors, or even the beautiful garnishes—although those all help. The real secret is in the syrups, cordials, and infusions that give every sip depth, complexity, and a unique twist.

Welcome to Mocktail Syrups and Flavors, Book 3 of the **Mocktails for Every Day series!** This book is dedicated to the art of flavor-making, giving you everything you need to create delicious homemade syrups, cordials, and infusions that will take your mocktails (and everyday drinks) to the next level. Whether you're crafting a refreshing summer spritz, a cozy winter warmer, or a sophisticated herbal infusion, these recipes will add layers of taste you simply can't get from store-bought options.

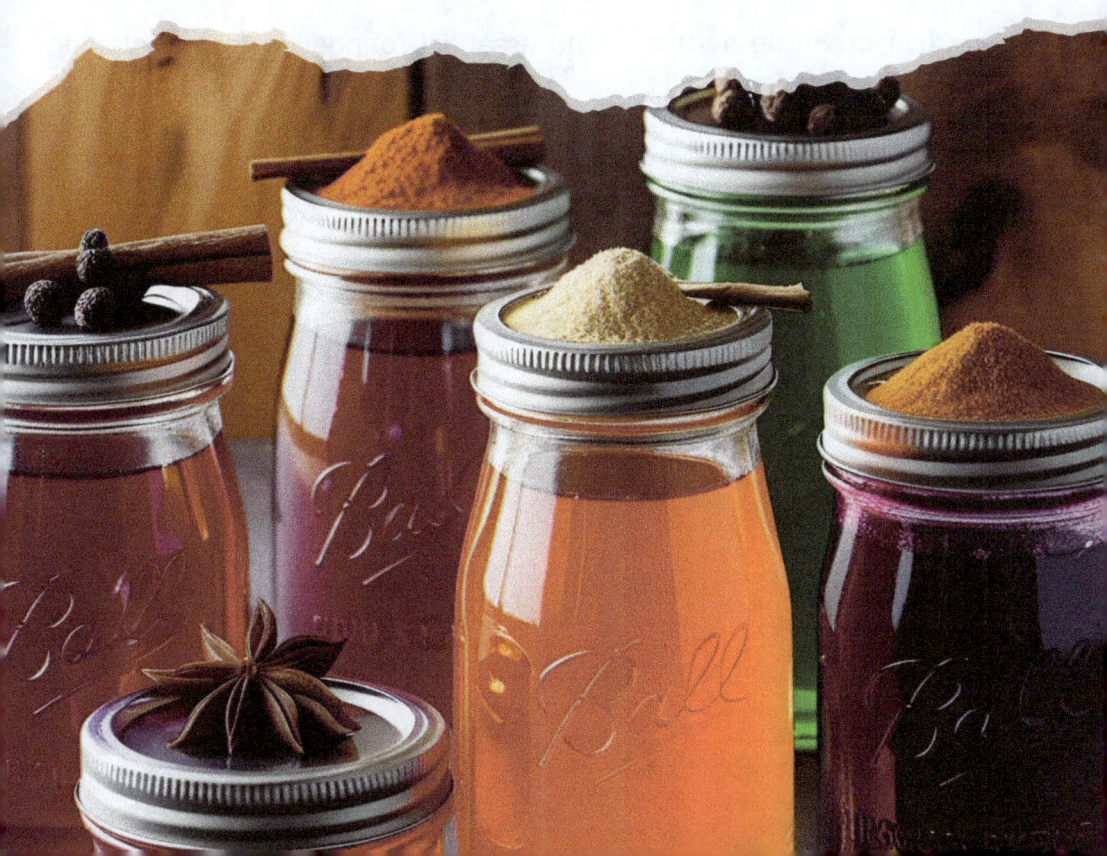

Why Make Your Own Syrups and Cordials?

If you've ever picked up a bottle of commercial flavored syrup, you've probably noticed a long list of preservatives, artificial flavors, and unnecessary additives. When you make your own, you control exactly what goes in—using real, fresh ingredients that taste better, are healthier, and give your drinks a richness that pre-made syrups just can't match. Plus, homemade syrups and infusions aren't just for mocktails! You can drizzle them over pancakes, stir them into coffee or tea, mix them into desserts, or even use them in marinades for an unexpected burst of flavor.

What You'll Find in This Book

This book is an amalgamation of all the syrup, cordial, and infusion recipes from the Mocktails for Every Day series, plus a few new surprises. We've even included the nut milk recipes from Winter Warmers, so you can make rich, creamy dairy alternatives to pair with your drinks.

Inside, you'll discover:

- **Classic simple syrups** – The essential foundation for sweetening and flavoring mocktails
- **Herbal and floral infusions** – Delicate, aromatic flavors from fresh herbs, teas, and edible flowers
- **Fruit-based cordials** – Bright, vibrant syrups bursting with fresh fruit goodness
- **Nut milks** – Perfect creamy additions for richer mocktails and warm drinks

How to Use This Book

Each recipe is designed to be simple, approachable, and versatile. While they were created with mocktails in mind, feel free to experiment—add a splash to sparkling water for an instant flavored soda, stir a spoonful into your morning tea, or even blend an infusion into a homemade salad dressing.

If you're following along with the **Mocktails for Every Day series**, this book serves as your go-to reference guide for all things syrup-related. Whether you're making a mocktail from one of our other books or inventing your own, you'll find endless inspiration here.

So grab your favorite ingredients, a saucepan, and a few bottles to store your homemade creations—it's time to elevate your drinks with incredible homemade flavors!

The Importance of Simple Syrups in Mocktail Making

Mocktails may be alcohol-free, but they should never be flavor-free. One of the easiest ways to add depth, balance, and complexity to a mocktail is through simple syrups. These humble sweeteners are the backbone of great drinks, providing a smooth consistency and a way to carry flavor evenly throughout the drink.

Whether you prefer classic sugar syrups, herbal infusions, or bold spiced variations, mastering the art of syrup-making will take your mocktails from ordinary to extraordinary.

Why Simple Syrups Matter

If you've ever added plain sugar to a cold drink, you've probably noticed how it sinks to the bottom without dissolving properly. That's where simple syrup comes in. By dissolving sugar in water beforehand, you create a liquid sweetener that blends seamlessly into any drink—hot or cold—ensuring even sweetness without any gritty texture.

But simple syrups do more than just sweeten. They:

- **Enhance flavors** – The right syrup can highlight the fruit, spice, or herb notes in a drink.
- **Balance acidity** – Many mocktails use citrus, which can be too tart without the right level of sweetness.
- **Carry aromatics** – Infused syrups allow you to introduce subtle flavors that would otherwise be lost.
- **Provide consistency** – A well-made syrup ensures a smooth, well-mixed mocktail without sugar settling at the bottom.

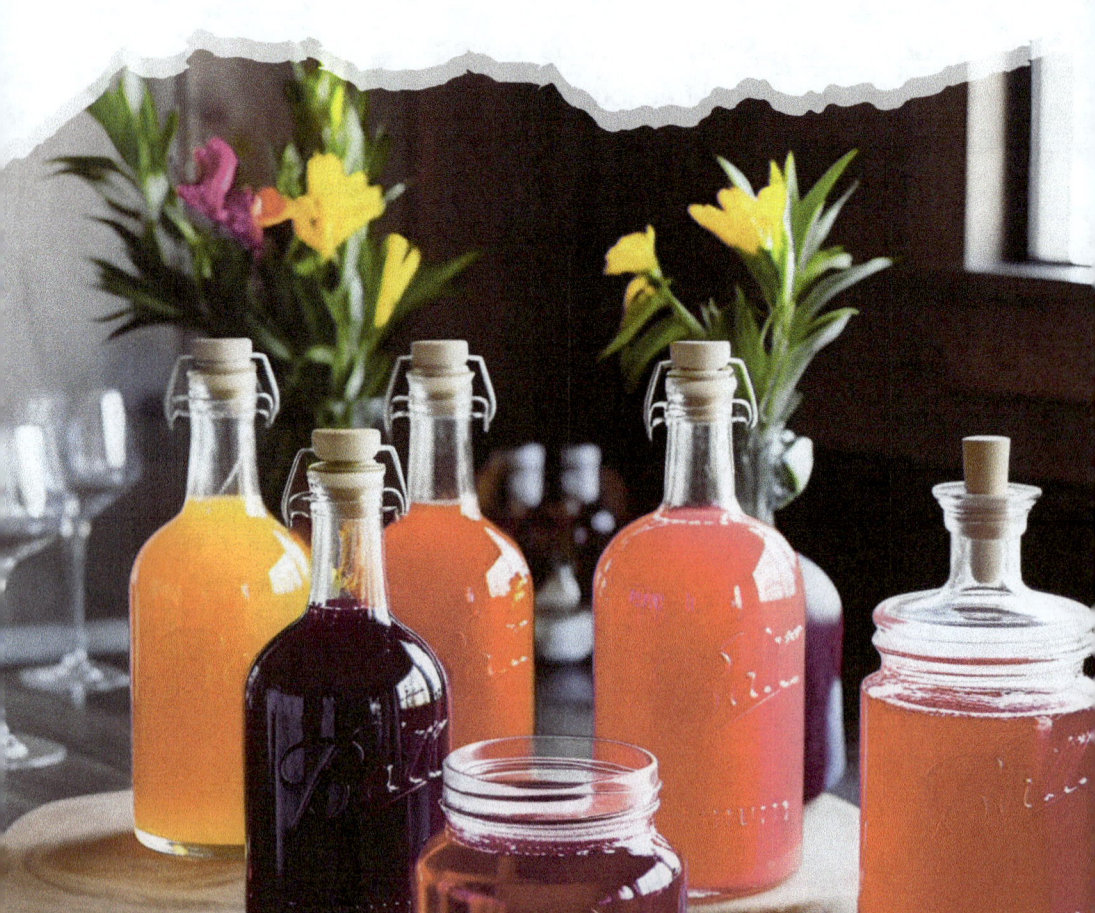

The Classic Simple Syrup Recipe

The foundation of all great syrups is a basic 1:1 simple syrup, which is just:

- 1 cup sugar
- 1 cup water

Simply combine the two in a saucepan over medium heat, stirring until the sugar is completely dissolved. Let it cool, then store it in a clean bottle or jar in the fridge for up to a month.

For a richer and more intense sweetness, try a 2:1 syrup (rich simple syrup) using:

- 2 cups sugar
- 1 cup water

This results in a thicker, more syrupy texture, which works beautifully in mocktails with bold flavors like coffee, dark berries, or warm spices.

Syrup vs. Cordial vs. Infusion

Feature	Cordial	Syrup	Infusion
Main Ingredients	Fruit juice, sugar, acid (sometimes herbs/spices)	Sugar and water with a single flavor	Water, alcohol, or oil with botanicals
Texture	Thicker than juice but thinner than syrup	Thick, viscous	Thin, like tea
Sweetness Level	Moderately sweet with tart balance	Very sweet	No sugar added
Common Uses	Mocktails, sodas, cooking, desserts	Mocktails, cocktails, coffee, tea	Tea, tinctures, flavored oils, spirits
Example	Lime cordial, elderflower cordial	Vanilla syrup, honey syrup	Chamomile infusion, mint tea

Creative Variations to Try

While this book contains a variety of tested and perfected syrup recipes, simple syrups are also a great place to experiment. Here are some fun variations to spark your creativity:

Citrusy Syrups
- Adding citrus zest or juice to a simple syrup can create bright, refreshing flavors:
- Lemon zest + honey syrup (pairs well with iced tea mocktails)
- Lime + coconut sugar syrup (great for tropical mocktails)
- Orange + vanilla bean syrup (delicious in winter warmers)

Herbal & Floral Infusions
- Infusing herbs and flowers into your syrup adds delicate aromatics:
- Basil simple syrup (perfect for summer spritzes)
- Rosemary + honey syrup (a great match for berry mocktails)
- Lavender + chamomile syrup (ideal for soothing evening drinks)

Spicy & Warm Syrups
- For a bold kick, try adding spices or heat:
- Cinnamon + star anise syrup (amazing in autumn and winter drinks)
- Ginger + turmeric syrup (great for zesty, warming mocktails)
- Jalapeño + honey syrup (adds a gentle heat to fruit-based mocktails)

Unique Sweeteners

Swapping out white sugar for other sweeteners creates a completely different profile:
- Maple syrup simple syrup – Adds richness and depth to nutty or warm drinks.
- Agave syrup + lime zest – A natural alternative that's perfect for citrus-based mocktails.
- Brown sugar + vanilla – Creates a caramel-like flavor that works beautifully in creamy mocktails.

Experimentation

While recipes are a great starting point, the best part of making mocktails is playing with flavors. Here are a few ways to get creative with your syrups:

- **Blend flavors** – Combine different herbs, fruits, and spices to create signature syrups.
- **Use seasonal ingredients** – Fresh berries in summer, cinnamon in winter—let the seasons guide your choices.
- **Adjust sweetness** – Prefer a lighter mocktail? Reduce the sugar ratio or mix syrups with herbal teas for a less sweet base.
- **Try unexpected pairings** – Cucumber + mint? Cardamom + pear? Don't be afraid to test out unique combinations!

Final Thoughts

Mastering simple syrups is the easiest way to elevate your mocktail game. Whether you stick with classic recipes or experiment with your own creations, these syrups will transform the way you approach drink-making.

So grab a saucepan, some fresh ingredients, and let your imagination run wild—your perfect signature mocktail might be just one syrup away!

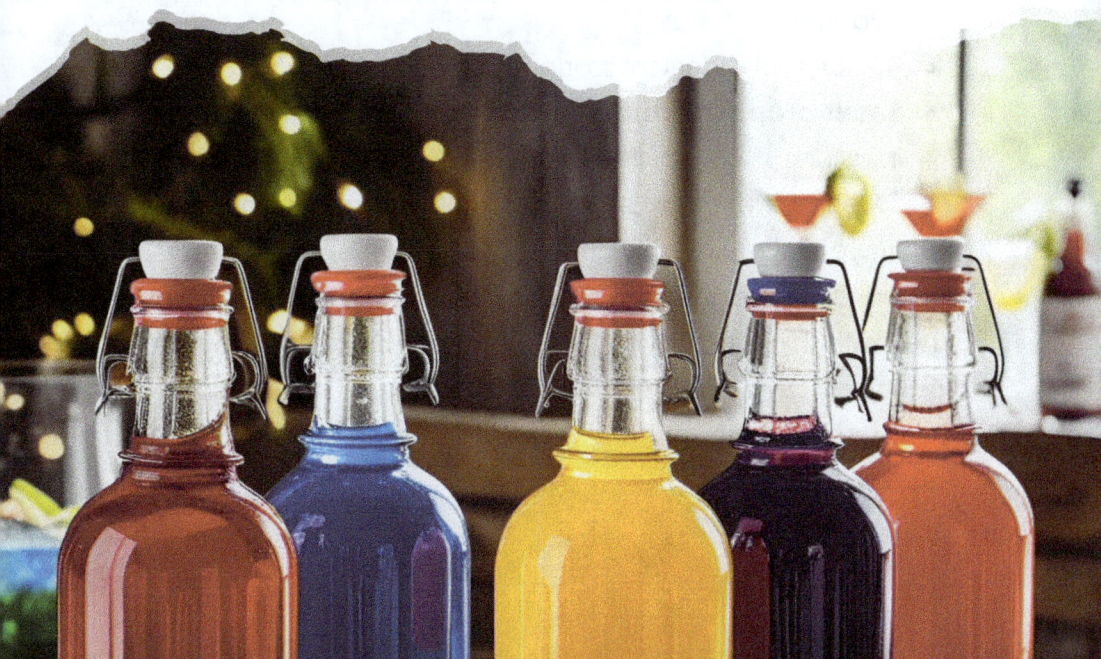

Tools & Equipment: Keeping It Simple

One of the best things about making syrups, cordials, and infusions is that you don't need fancy equipment or specialized tools. In fact, you probably already have everything you need in your kitchen. Unlike complex cooking techniques that require precision instruments, syrup-making is forgiving, flexible, and beginner-friendly.

With just a few basic tools, you can create incredible flavors that will take your mocktails (and everyday drinks) to the next level.

Essential Tools for Easy Syrup & Cordial Making

- **Saucepan:** A small to medium-sized heavy-bottomed saucepan is ideal for making syrups. If you're making larger batches, a bigger pot can help prevent spills when stirring.
- **Stirring Spoon:** A simple wooden spoon or silicone spatula works perfectly for dissolving sugar and stirring ingredients while they simmer.
- **Jars & Bottles for Storage:** You'll need clean, airtight bottles or jars to store your syrups and cordials. Glass is best because it won't absorb flavors and is easy to sterilize.
    - **Swing-top bottles** – Great for cordials and syrups you'll use frequently.
    - **Mason jars** – Ideal for storing smaller batches.
    - **Small dropper bottles** – Perfect for concentrated extracts and infusions.
- **Fine Mesh Strainer or Cheesecloth:** If you're using herbs, spices, or fruit in your syrups, you'll need to strain out the solids before storing. A fine-mesh strainer works well, but for very fine particles, a cheesecloth or nut milk bag will give you a crystal-clear syrup.
- **Ice Cube Trays (For Freezing Syrups):** Syrups freeze beautifully, and using an ice cube tray allows you to portion out small amounts for future use.

- **Funnel:** A small funnel helps you transfer your syrup into bottles cleanly without spills or waste.
- **Measuring Cups & Spoons:** While syrup-making is not an exact science, having basic measuring tools helps ensure balanced flavors and consistency.

Storing & Preserving Your Syrups, Cordials & Infusions

Since homemade syrups don't contain preservatives like commercial products, they have a shorter shelf life. However, with proper storage, you can keep them fresh for weeks.

Refrigerator Storage (Short-Term)

Most simple syrups, cordials, and infusions will keep for 2-4 weeks in the fridge, depending on the ingredients used.

- **Basic sugar syrups (1:1 ratio)** – Last about 2 weeks in a sealed container.
- **Rich syrups (2:1 sugar-to-water ratio)** – Last about a month due to the higher sugar content.
- **Infused syrups (with herbs, fruit, or spices)** – Best used within 1-2 weeks for the freshest flavor.

Pro Tip: Always use a clean, dry spoon when scooping syrup out of a jar to avoid contamination!

Freezing Syrups (For Long-Term Storage)

Freezing is the easiest way to preserve syrups for months while keeping them fresh.

- **Pour syrup into ice cube trays** – This allows you to pop out small portions as needed.
- **Transfer frozen cubes into a zip-lock bag or airtight container** – Label with the date and flavor.
- Use within 3-6 months for best quality.

How to Use Frozen Syrup: Simply thaw a cube in the fridge overnight or pop it straight into hot tea for instant flavor!

Preserving Infusions & Cordials

If you want to make your cordials and infusions last longer, you can:

- **Increase the sugar content** – A higher sugar ratio acts as a natural preservative.
- **Use citrus juice (like lemon) or citric acid** – This helps extend shelf life and adds a fresh zing.
- **Store in sterilized glass bottles** – Running bottles through boiling water before use helps prevents spoilage.

Final Thoughts: Keep It Fun & Simple!

Making your own syrups, cordials, and infusions is easy, inexpensive, and endlessly customizable. With just a few basic tools and simple storage tricks, you can have a flavor arsenal ready to elevate any mocktail—or even your morning coffee!

So grab a saucepan, get creative, and start crafting your own signature flavors!

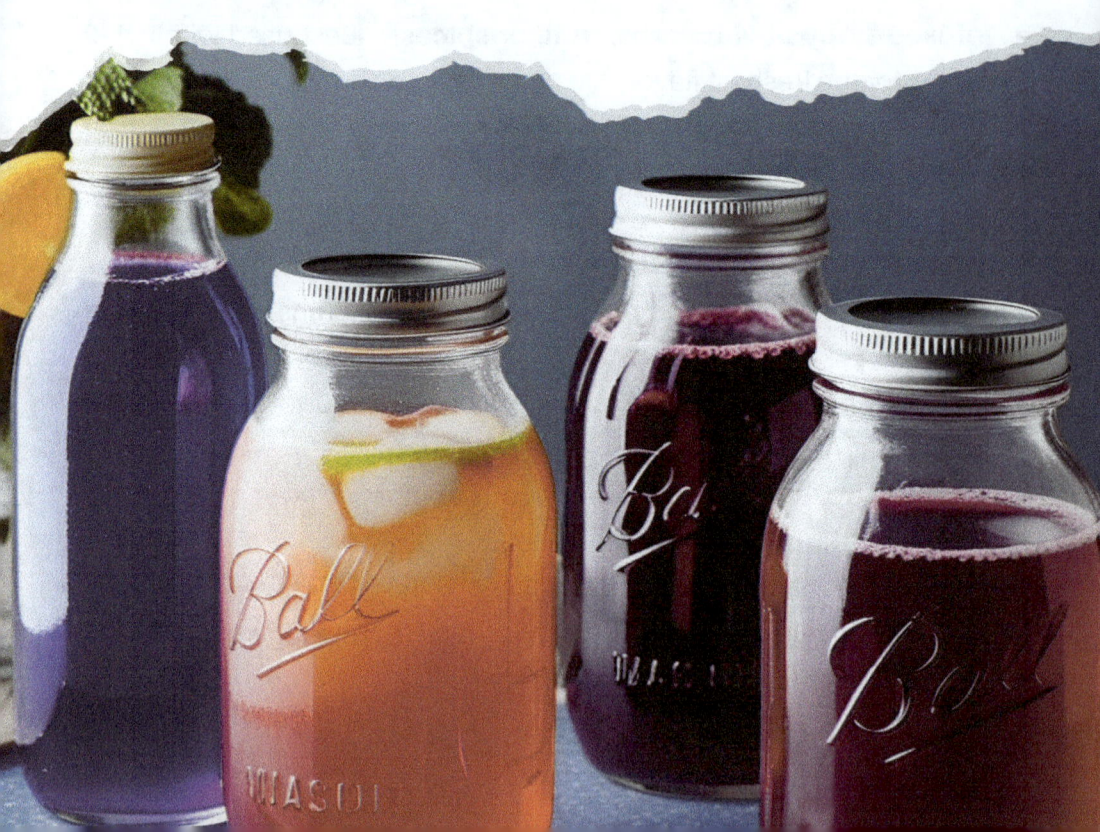

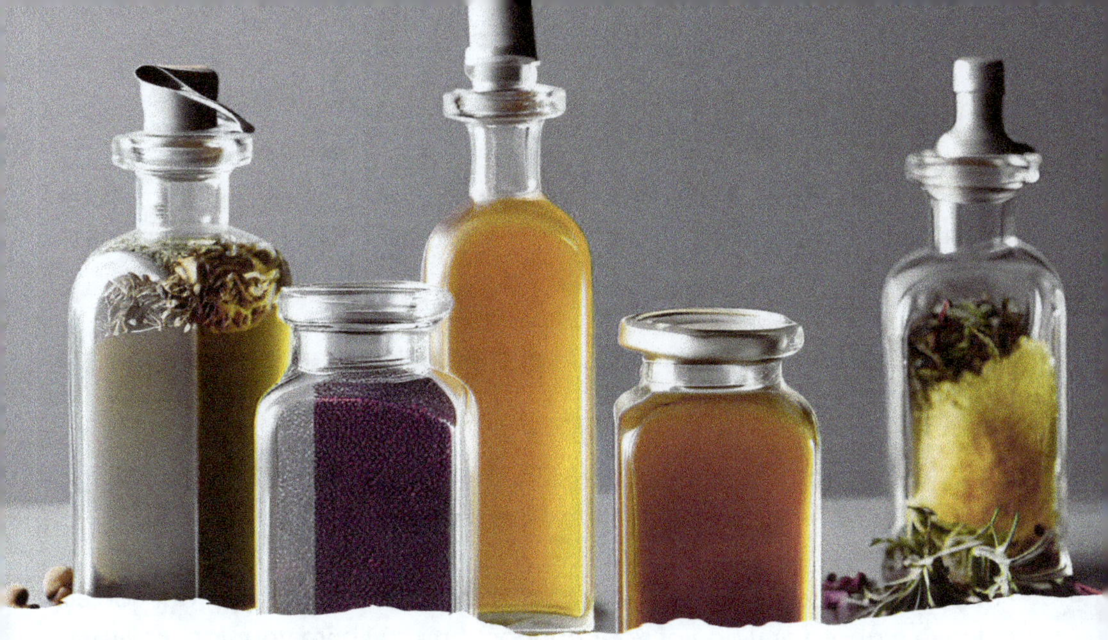

SIMPLE SYRUPS

These essential syrups provide sweetness and depth, making them the perfect starting point for crafting balanced and flavorful drinks.

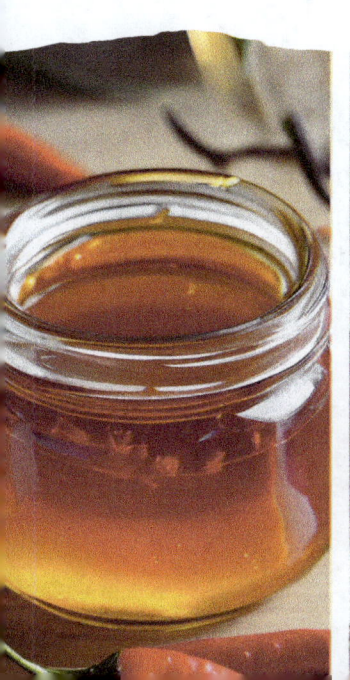 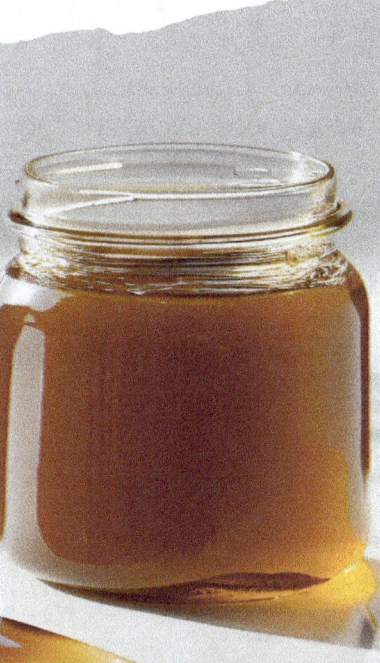 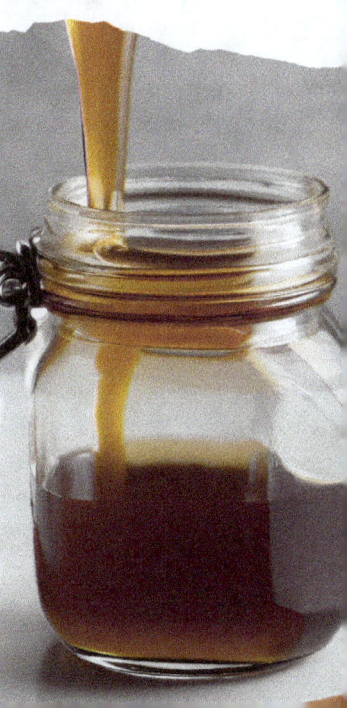

What is a simple syrup?

All of these recipes are based on a simple syrup made from 1 cup of water and 1 cup of granulated sugar, with the addition of different flavor base ingredients.

They will make enough syrup for several cocktails and will keep in the fridge for a couple of weeks.

If you wanted to experiment, by making your own flavored syrups that are not included here, you could follow the proportions in these recipes.

Follow the QR code in this book to reach our website and join our socials to leave a photo or video of your concoctions, to share your ideas with all our readers, and see what ideas others have come up with.

The Magic of Syrups: Elevating Your Mocktails

A great mocktail isn't just about replacing alcohol—it's about balancing flavors, creating depth, and crafting something truly special. And one of the best ways to achieve this is by using homemade syrups. These flavorful additions give your drinks body, sweetness, and complexity, transforming simple ingredients into something extraordinary.

Why Make Your Own Syrups?

Store-bought syrups can be convenient, but they're often loaded with preservatives, artificial flavors, and excessive sugar. When you make your own, you control everything—the sweetness, the intensity, and the quality of ingredients. Whether you want a bright citrus syrup, a rich spiced blend, or a floral-infused delight, homemade syrups let you craft unique flavors tailored to your taste.

The Key to Balance
In mixology, whether alcoholic or alcohol-free, a balanced drink is key. Syrups help by adding:
- Sweetness – to counteract acidity from citrus or bitterness from certain ingredients.
- Body & Mouthfeel – making drinks feel more luxurious and satisfying.
- Depth of Flavor – from rich caramel notes to herbal, spiced, or floral layers.

Essential Syrup-Making Tips
Making syrups at home is surprisingly simple, but a few key techniques will help you get the best results:
- Use Fresh Ingredients where possible– Fresh fruits, herbs, and spices make a world of difference.
- Keep the Heat Low – Simmer gently to extract flavors without burning or overcooking.
- Strain Thoroughly – A fine mesh strainer or cheesecloth ensures a smooth, clean syrup.
- Experiment with Infusions – Steeping herbs, teas, or spices can add unexpected depth.
- Store Properly – Keep syrups refrigerated in a sealed glass bottle for freshness. Discard if they become cloudy or smell 'off'. Alternatvely, freezing in ice cube molds then decanting into a sealed, labeled and dated bag, allows longer storage.

How to Use Syrups in Mocktails
Once you've made your syrups, the possibilities are endless! Here are some easy ways to use them:
- Classic Sweeteners – Swap out plain sugar or honey in any drink.
- Layered Flavors – Combine fruit, herbal, or spiced syrups for unique taste profiles.
- Flavored Sparkling Waters – Add a splash of syrup to soda water for a quick, refreshing drink.
- Coffee & Tea Enhancers – Try vanilla, cinnamon, or cardamom syrup in lattes and iced teas.
- Dessert Drizzles – Use leftover syrups over pancakes, ice cream, or yogurt.

Whether you're making a bright, tangy berry syrup or a rich, velvety caramel infusion, homemade syrups open the door to limitless creativity. In the next section, we'll dive into must-try syrup recipes to elevate your mocktails from good to unforgettable.

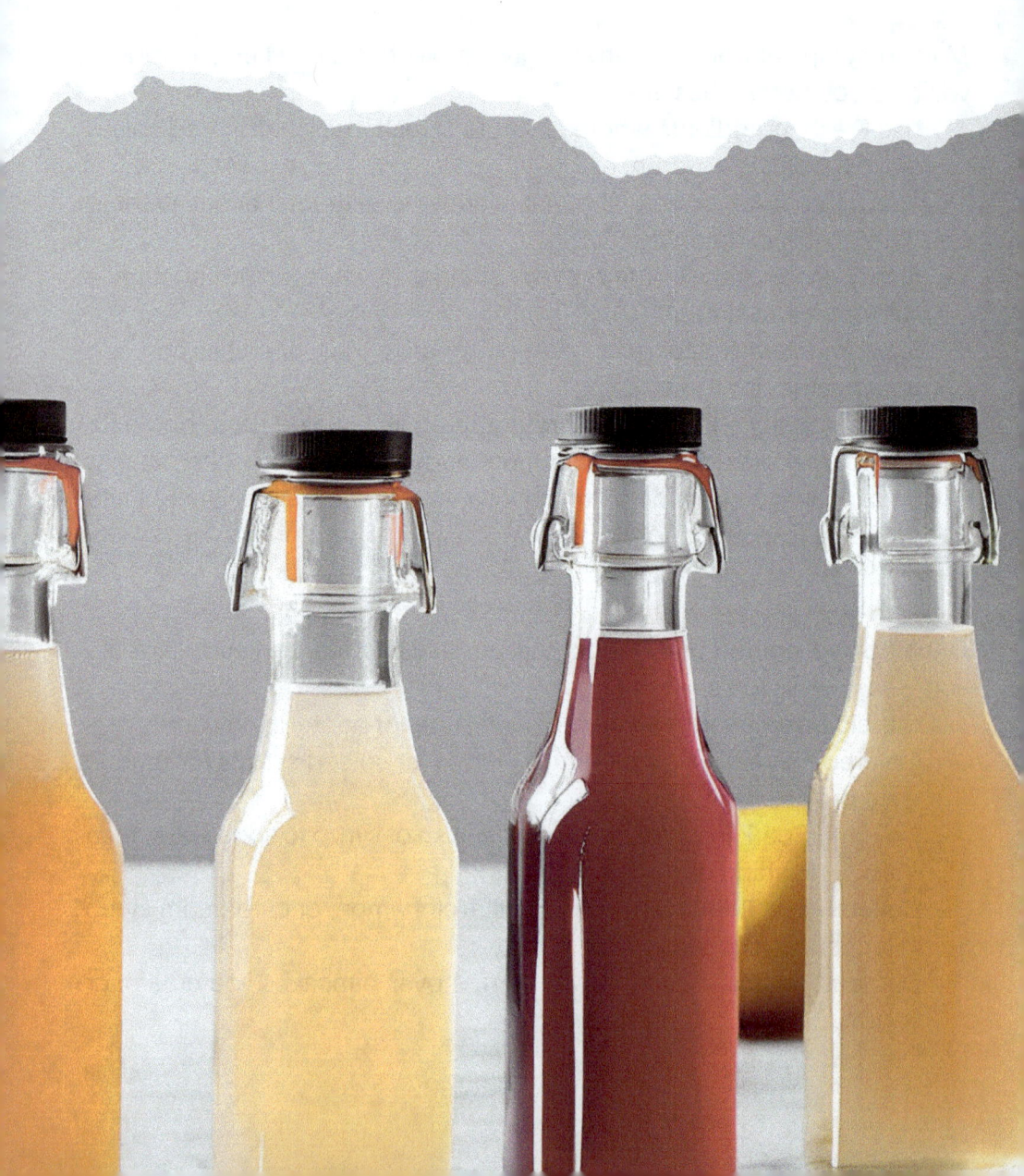

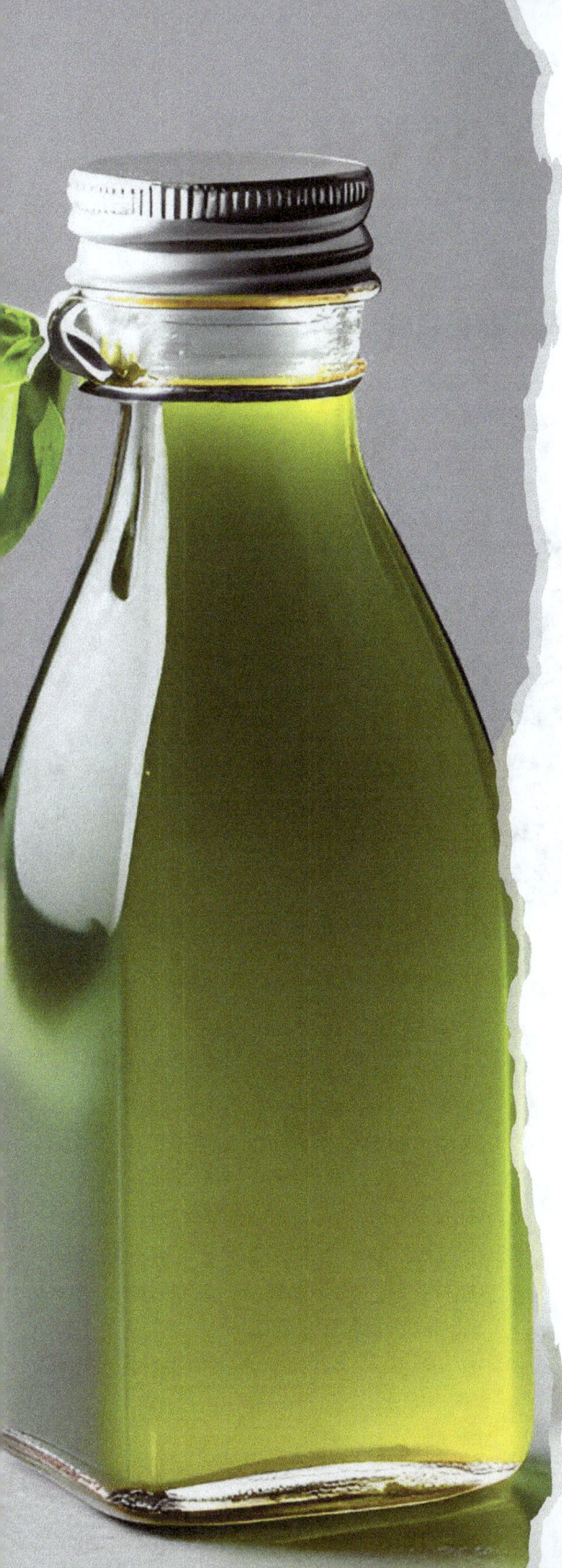

BASIL SYRUP

Ingredients

- 1 cup water
- 1 cup granulated sugar
- 1 cup fresh basil leaves

Procedure

1. In a saucepan, combine water, sugar, and basil leaves. Bring to a boil, then reduce the heat and simmer for 5 minutes.
2. Remove from heat and let the syrup steep for 15 minutes.
3. Strain out the basil leaves and let the syrup cool before pouring into a sterilized bottle or jar.
4. Store in the refrigerator for up to 2 weeks.

BERRY SYRUP

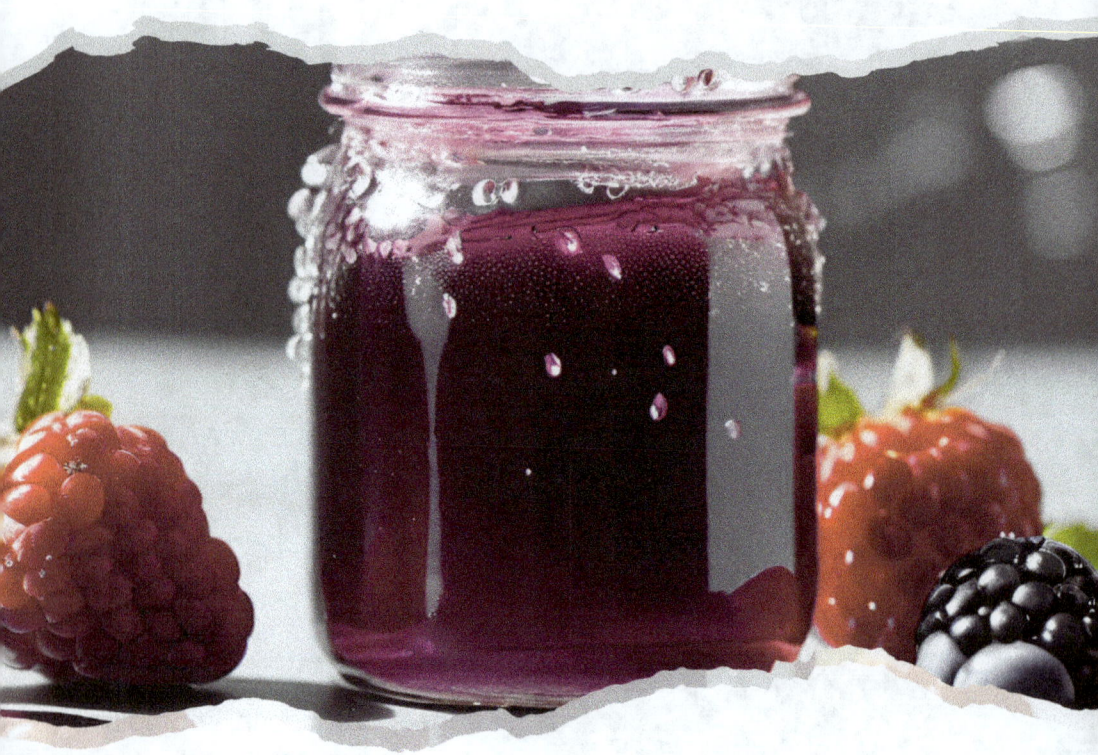

Ingredients

- 1 cup water
- 1 cup mixed berries (strawberries, raspberries, blueberries)
- 1 cup granulated sugar

Procedure

1. In a saucepan, combine the mixed berries, water, and sugar. Bring to a boil, then reduce the heat and simmer for 10 minutes until the berries break down.
2. Strain the mixture through a fine mesh sieve to remove the solids. Let the syrup cool before pouring into a sterilized bottle or jar.
3. Store in the refrigerator for up to 2 weeks.

CHILI-INFUSED SYRUP

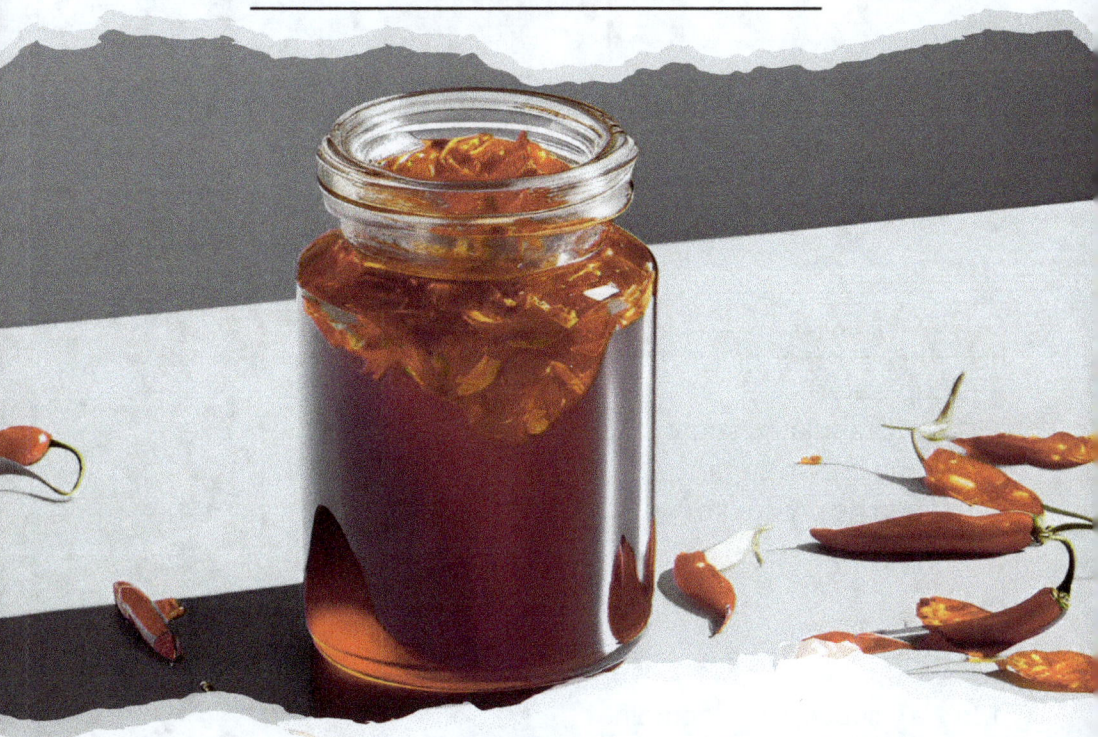

Ingredients

- 1 cup water
- 1 cup granulated sugar
- 1 fresh chili pepper, sliced

Procedure

1. In a saucepan, combine water, sugar, and chili slices. Bring to a boil, then reduce the heat and simmer for 5 minutes.
2. Remove from heat and let the syrup steep for 10 15 minutes, depending on how spicy you like it.
3. Strain out the chili slices and let the syrup cool before pouring into a sterilized bottle or jar.
4. Store in the refrigerator for up to 2 weeks.

CARAMEL SYRUP

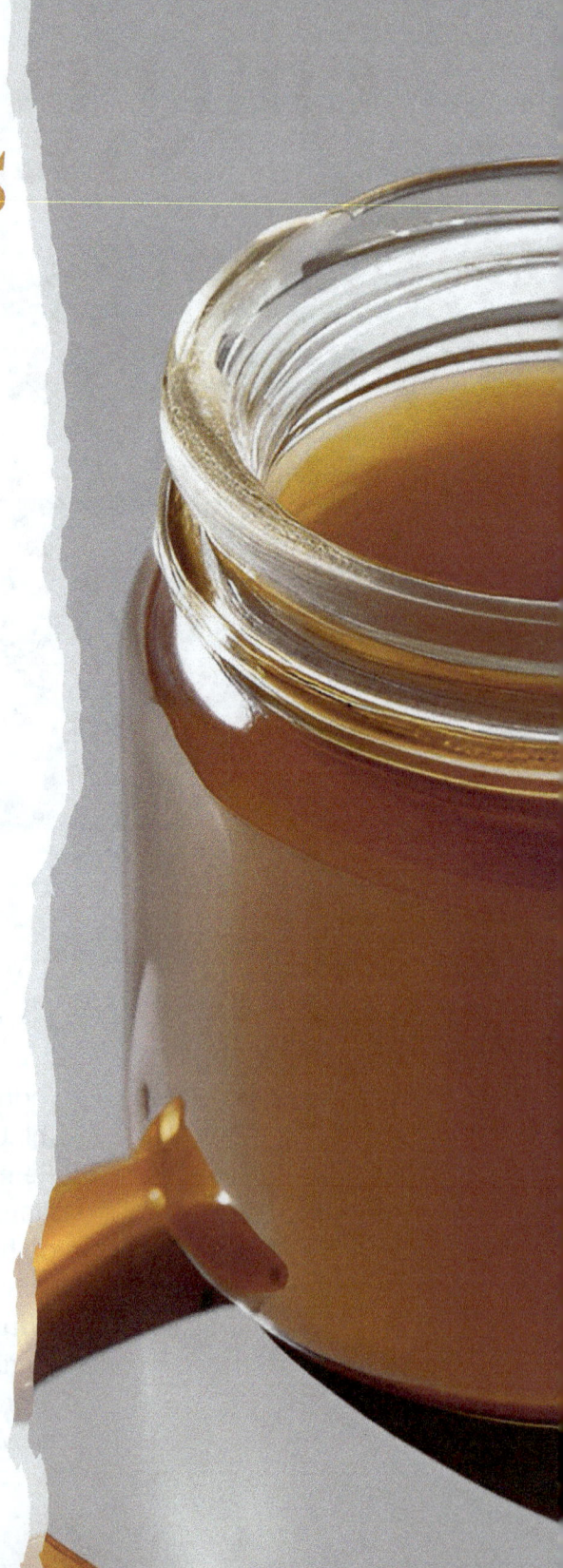

Ingredients

- 1 cup water
- 1 cup granulated sugar
- 1/2 cup brown sugar
- 1/4 cup heavy cream

Procedure

1. In a saucepan, combine water, granulated sugar, and brown sugar. Bring to a boil, then reduce the heat and simmer for 10 minutes.
2. Remove from heat, then slowly stir in the cream. Let the syrup cool before before pouring into a sterilized bottle or jar.
3. Store in the refrigerator for up to 2 weeks.

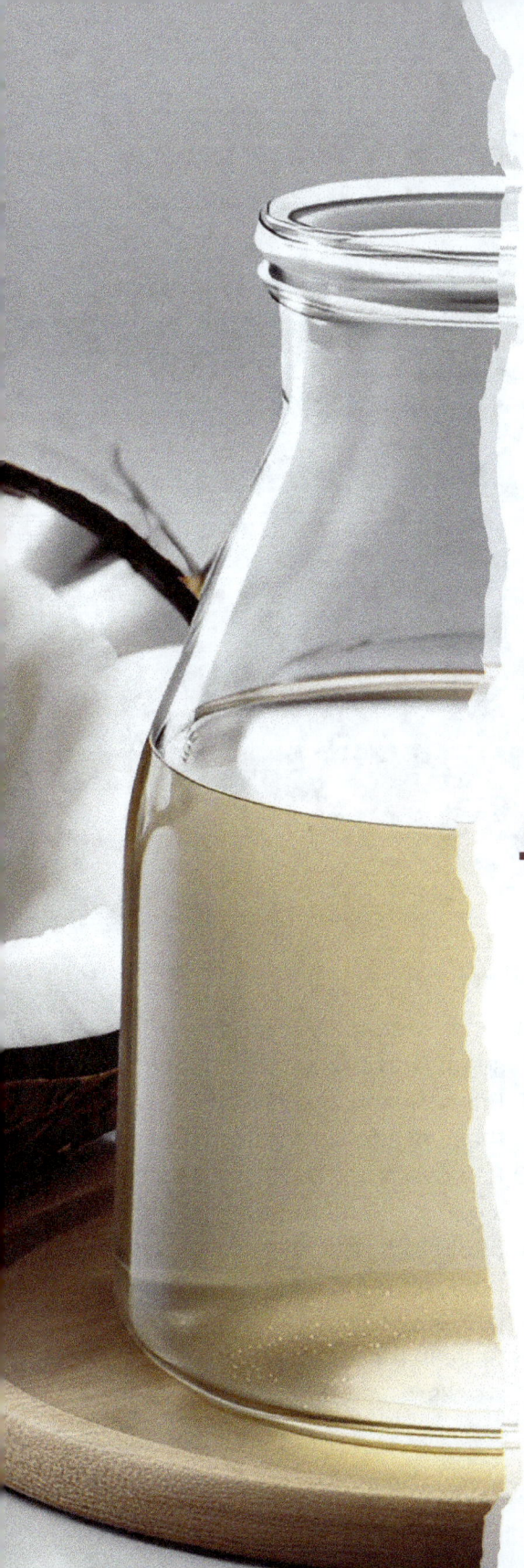

COCONUT SYRUP

Ingredients

- 1 cup water
- 1 cup granulated sugar
- 1/2 cup coconut milk

Procedure

1. In a saucepan, combine water, sugar, and coconut milk. Bring to a boil, then
2. reduce the heat and simmer for 5 minutes.
3. Remove from heat and let the syrup cool before pouring into a sterilized bottle or jar.
4. Store in the refrigerator for up to 2 weeks.

CINNAMON SYRUP

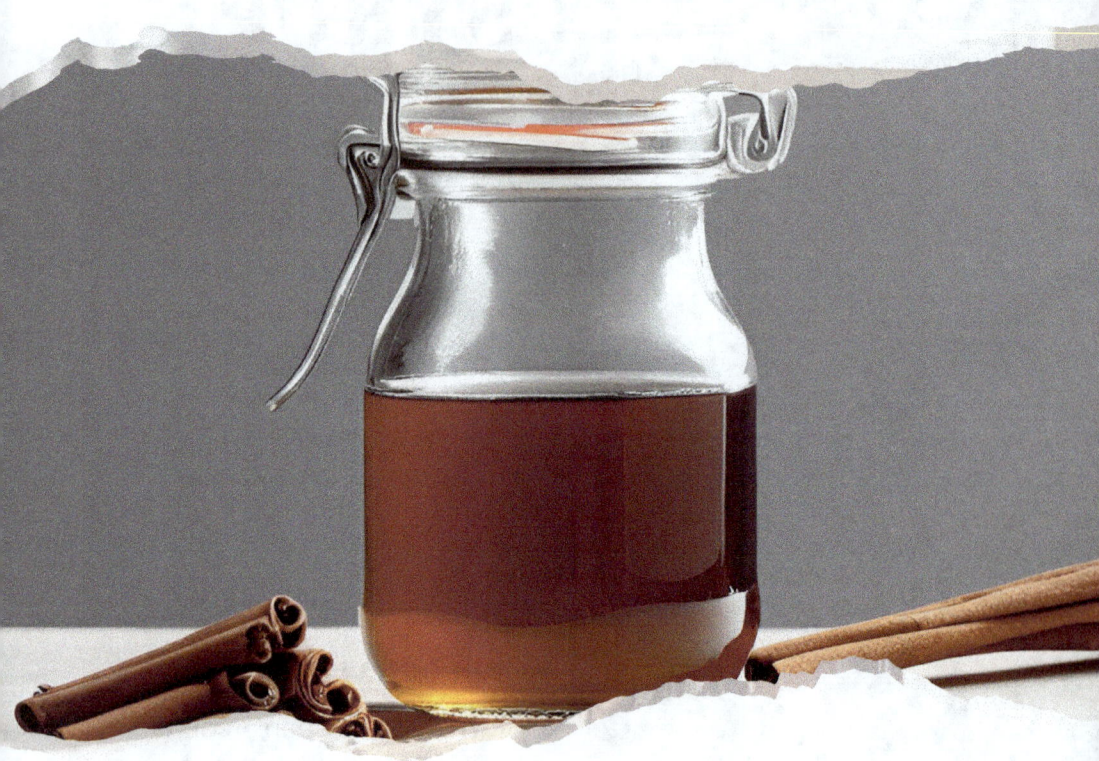

Ingredients

- 1 cup water
- 1 cup granulated sugar
- 3 cinnamon sticks

Procedure

1. In a saucepan, combine the water, sugar, and cinnamon sticks.
2. Bring the mixture to a boil, then reduce the heat and simmer for 10 minutes.
3. Remove from heat and let the syrup steep for 15 minutes.
4. Strain out the cinnamon sticks and pour the syrup into a sterilized bottle or jar.
5. Store in the refrigerator for up to 2 weeks.

CHOCOLATE SYRUP

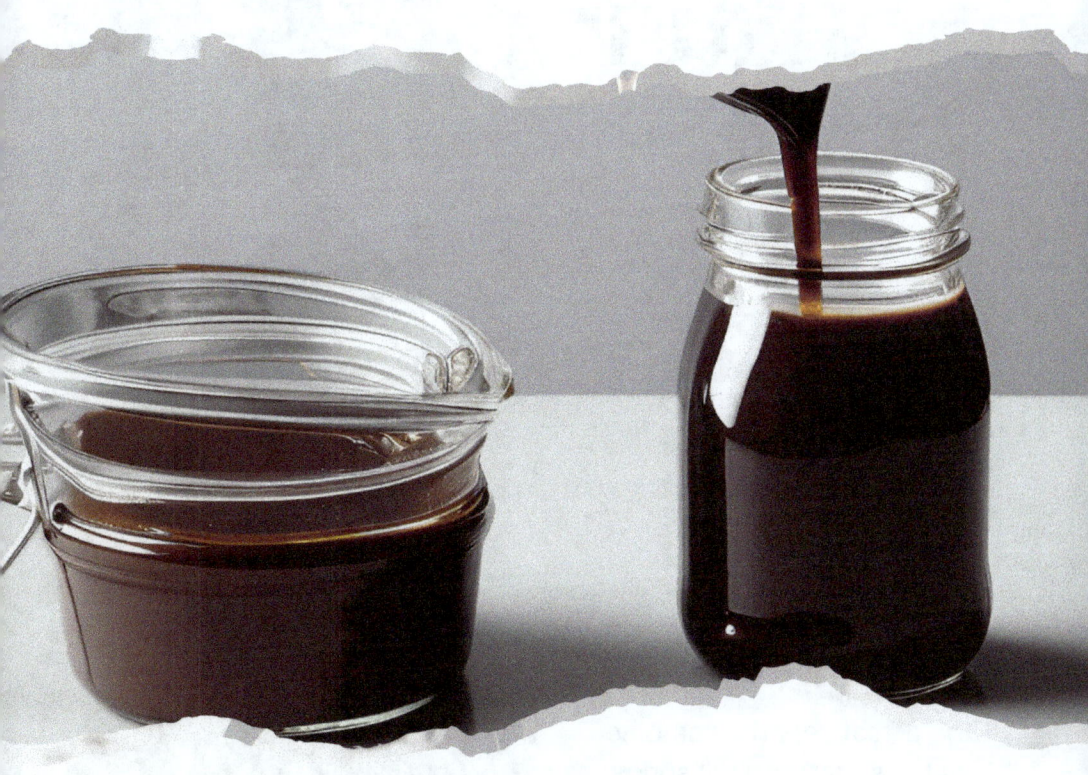

Ingredients

- 1 cup water
- 1 cup granulated sugar
- 1/2 cup cocoa powder
- 1 teaspoon vanilla extract

Procedure

1. In a saucepan, combine water, sugar, and cocoa powder. Bring to a boil, then reduce the heat and simmer for 5 minutes, stirring constantly.
2. Remove from heat and stir in the vanilla extract. Let the syrup cool before pouring into a sterilized bottle or jar.
3. Store in the refrigerator for up to 2 weeks.

DILL SYRUP

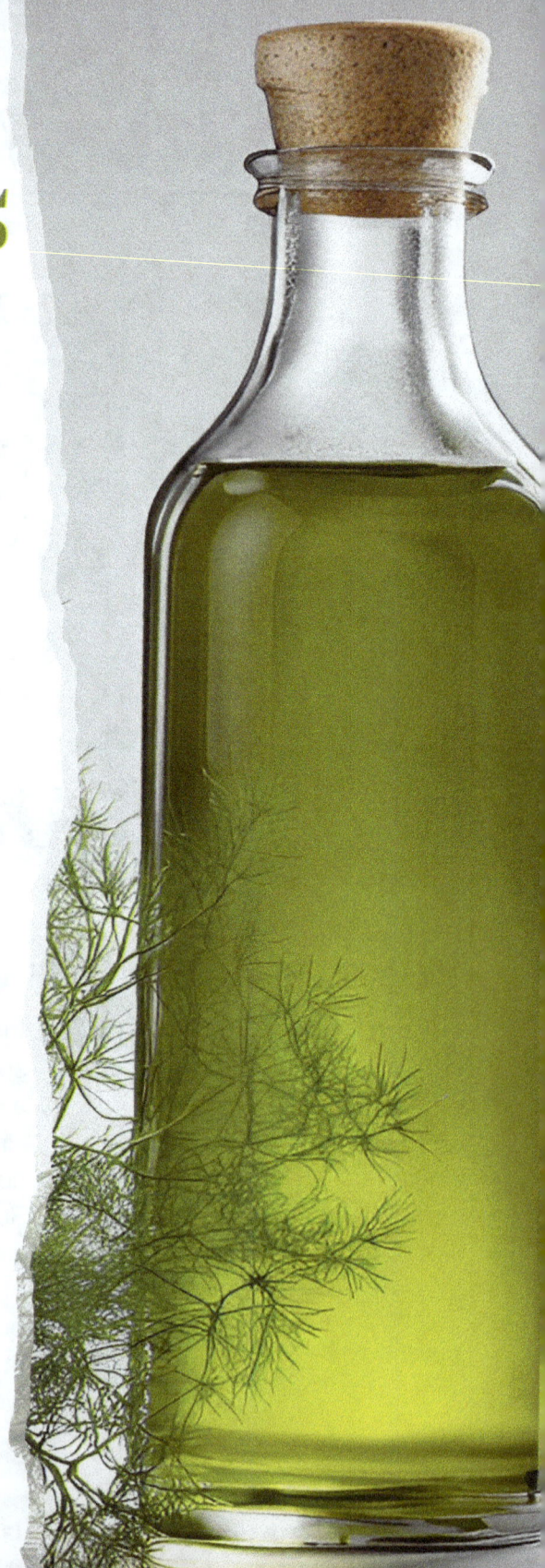

Ingredients

- 1 cup water
- 1 cup granulated sugar
- 1/2 cup fresh dill sprigs

Procedure

1. In a saucepan, combine water, sugar, and dill sprigs. Bring to a boil, then reduce the heat and simmer for 5 minutes.
2. Remove from heat and let the syrup steep for 15 minutes.
3. Strain out the dill and let the syrup cool before pouring into a sterilized bottle or jar.
4. Store in the refrigerator for up to 2 weeks.

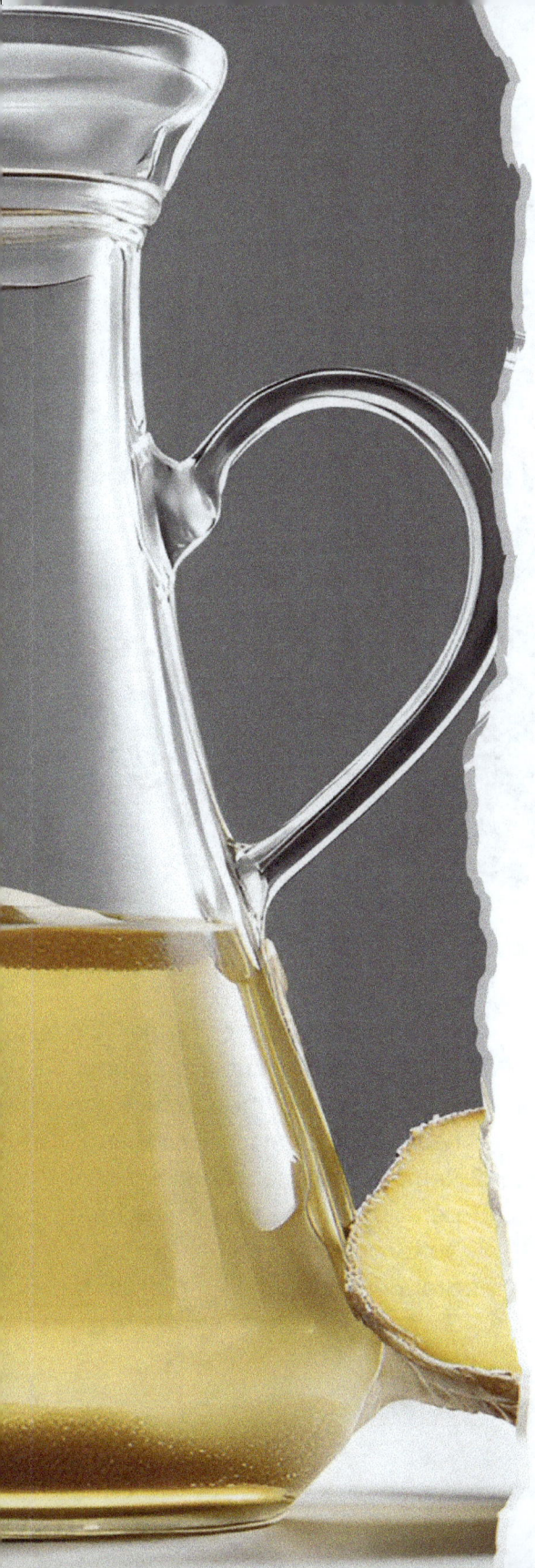

GINGER SYRUP

Ingredients

- 1 cup water
- 1 cup granulated sugar
- 1/2 cup fresh ginger root, sliced

Procedure

1. In a saucepan, combine the water, sugar, and ginger slices.
2. Bring the mixture to a boil, then reduce the heat and simmer for 10 minutes.
3. Remove from heat and let the syrup steep for 15 minutes.
4. Strain out the ginger slices and pour the syrup into a sterilized bottle or jar.
5. Store in the refrigerator for up to 2 weeks.

GRENADINE SYRUP

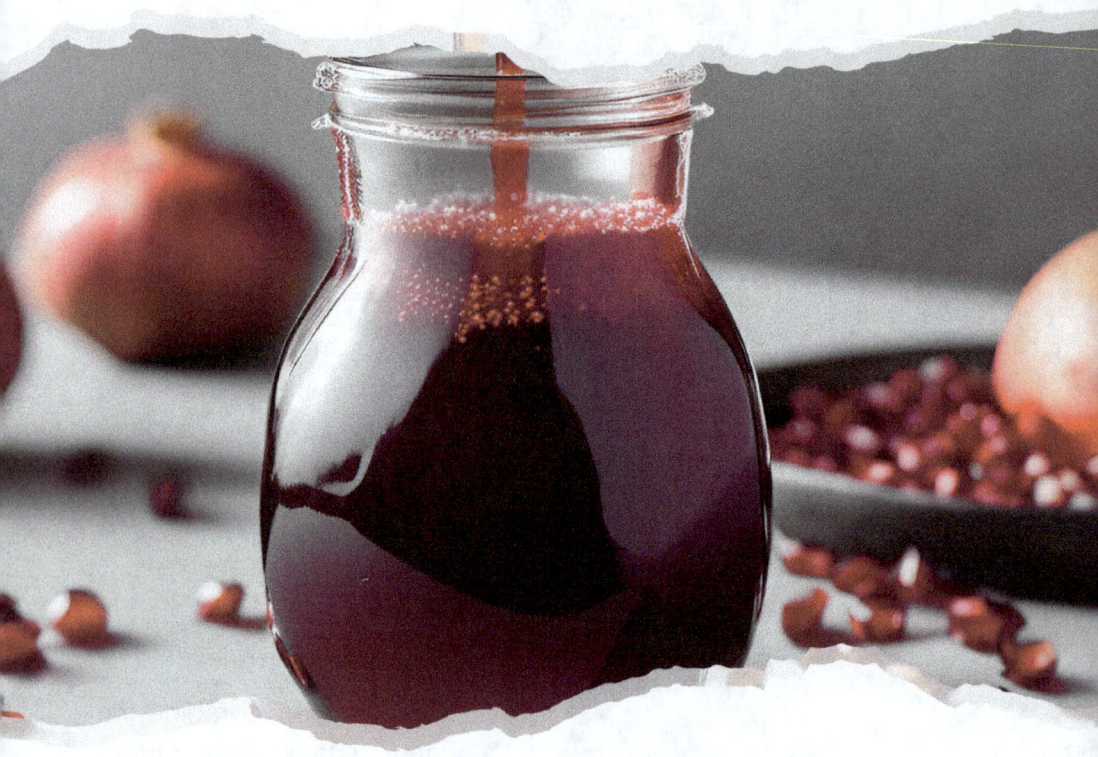

Ingredients

- 1 cup fresh pomegranate juice (from about 2 large pomegranates)
- 1 cup granulated sugar

Procedure

1. In a saucepan, combine the pomegranate juice and sugar. Bring to a boil, then reduce the heat and simmer for 5 minutes.
2. Remove from heat and let it cool before pouring into a sterilized bottle or jar.
3. Store in the refrigerator for up to 2 weeks.

HONEY SYRUP

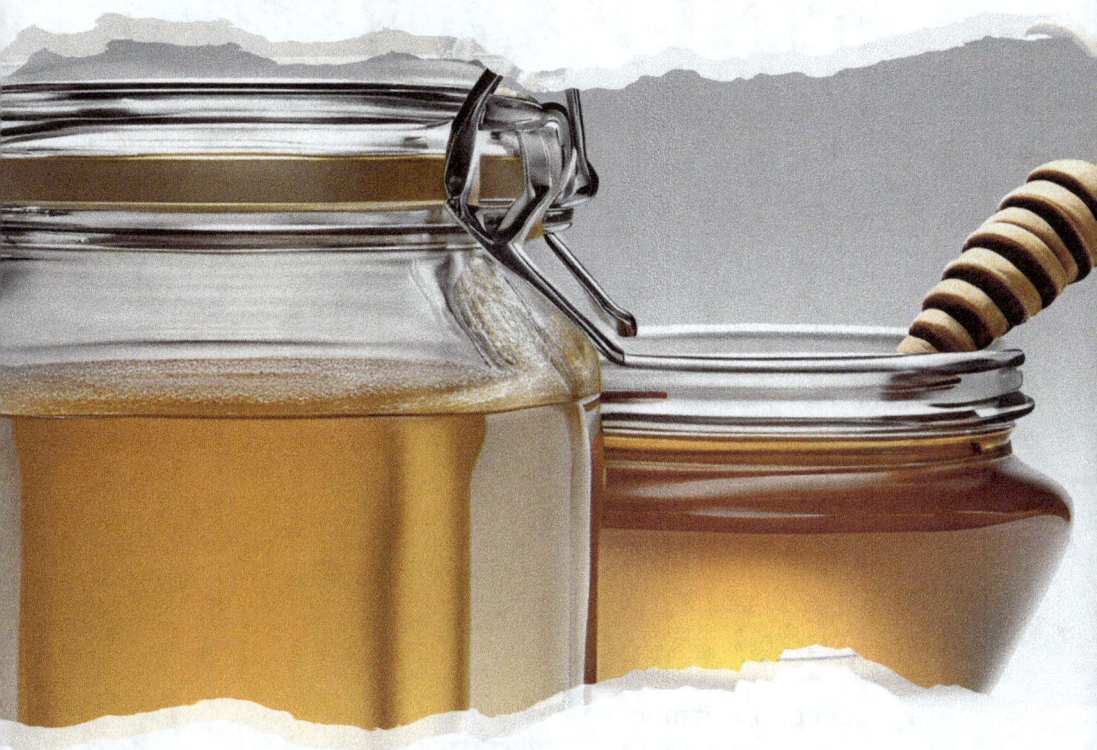

Ingredients

- 1/2 cup water
- 1/2 cup honey

Procedure

1. In a saucepan, combine honey and water. Heat over low heat, stirring until the honey dissolves completely.
2. Remove from heat and let the syrup cool before pouring into a sterilized bottle or jar.
3. Store in the refrigerator for up to 2 weeks.

HIBISCUS SYRUP

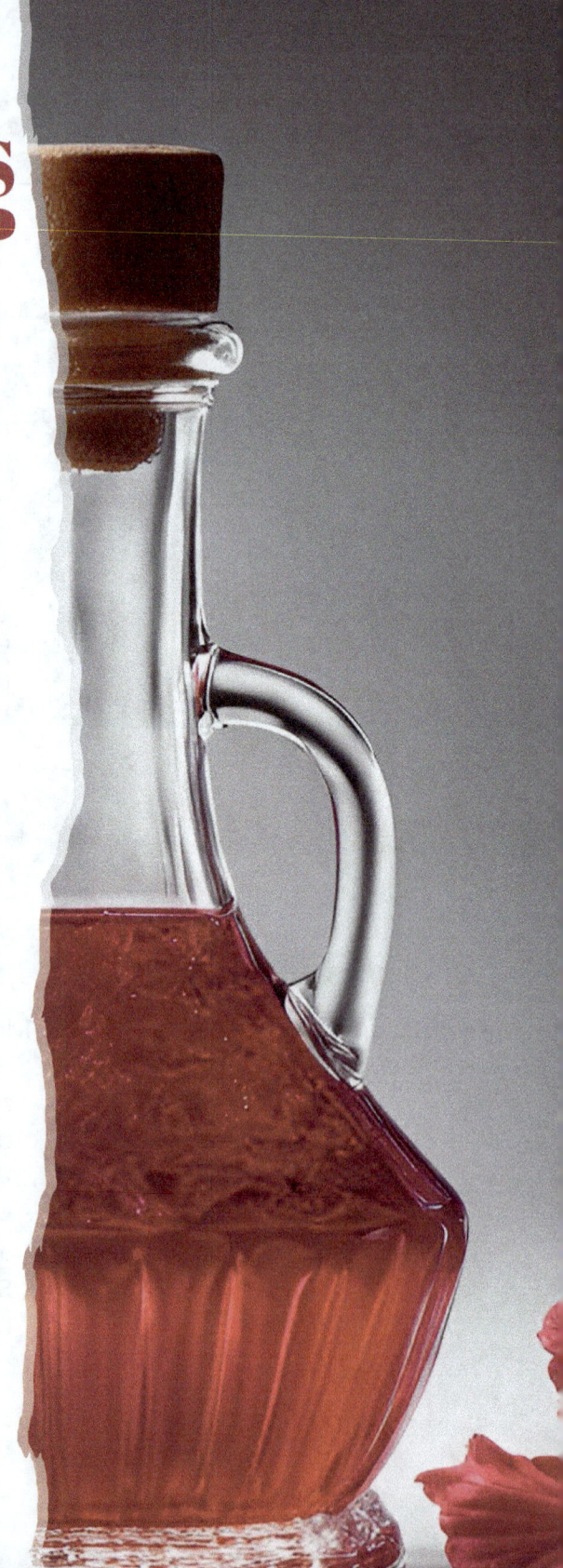

Ingredients

- 1 cup water
- 1 cup granulated sugar
- 1/2 cup dried hibiscus flowers

Procedure

1. In a saucepan, combine water, sugar, and hibiscus flowers. Bring to a boil, then reduce the heat and simmer for 5 minutes.
2. Remove from heat and let the syrup steep for 15 minutes. Strain out the hibiscus flowers and let the syrup cool before pouring into a sterilized bottle or jar.
3. Store in the refrigerator for up to 2 weeks.

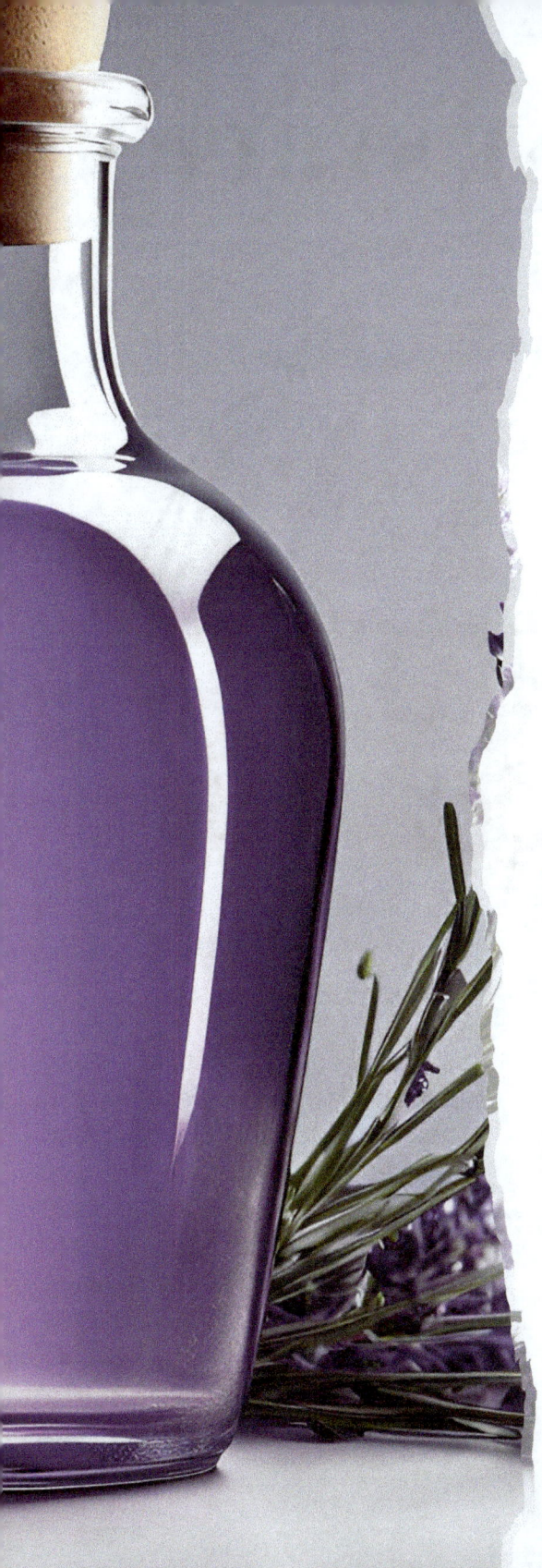

LAVENDER SYRUP

Ingredients

- 1 cup water
- 1 cup granulated sugar
- 2 tablespoons dried lavender flowers (food-grade)

Procedure

1. In a saucepan, combine water, sugar, and lavender flowers. Bring to a boil, then reduce the heat and simmer for 5 minutes.
2. Remove from heat and let the syrup steep for 15 minutes.
3. Strain out the lavender flowers and let the syrup cool before pouring into a sterilized bottle or jar.
4. Store in the refrigerator for up to 2 weeks.

JASMINE SYRUP

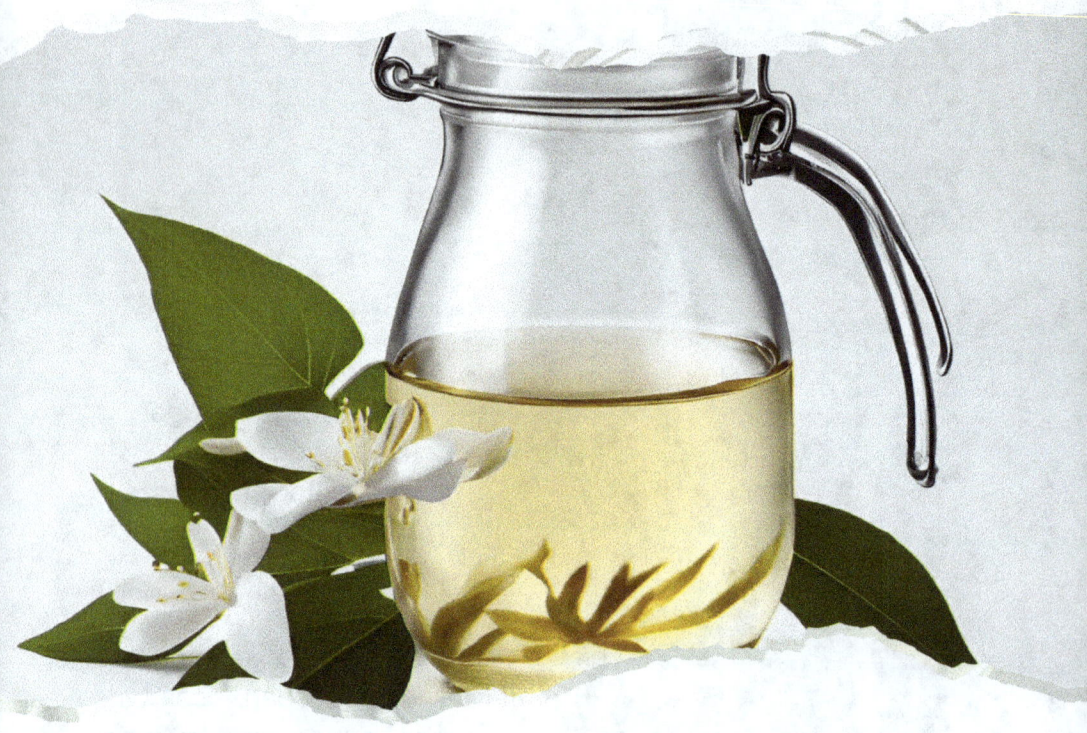

Ingredients

- 1 cup water
- 1 cup granulated sugar
- 2 tablespoons dried jasmine flowers (organic and food-grade)

Procedure

1. In a saucepan, combine water, sugar, and jasmine flowers. Bring to a boil, then reduce the heat and simmer for 5 minutes.
2. Remove from heat and let the syrup steep for 15 minutes. Strain out the jasmine flowers and let the syrup cool before pouring into a sterilized bottle or jar.
3. Store in the refrigerator for up to 2 weeks.

LEMONGRASS SYRUP

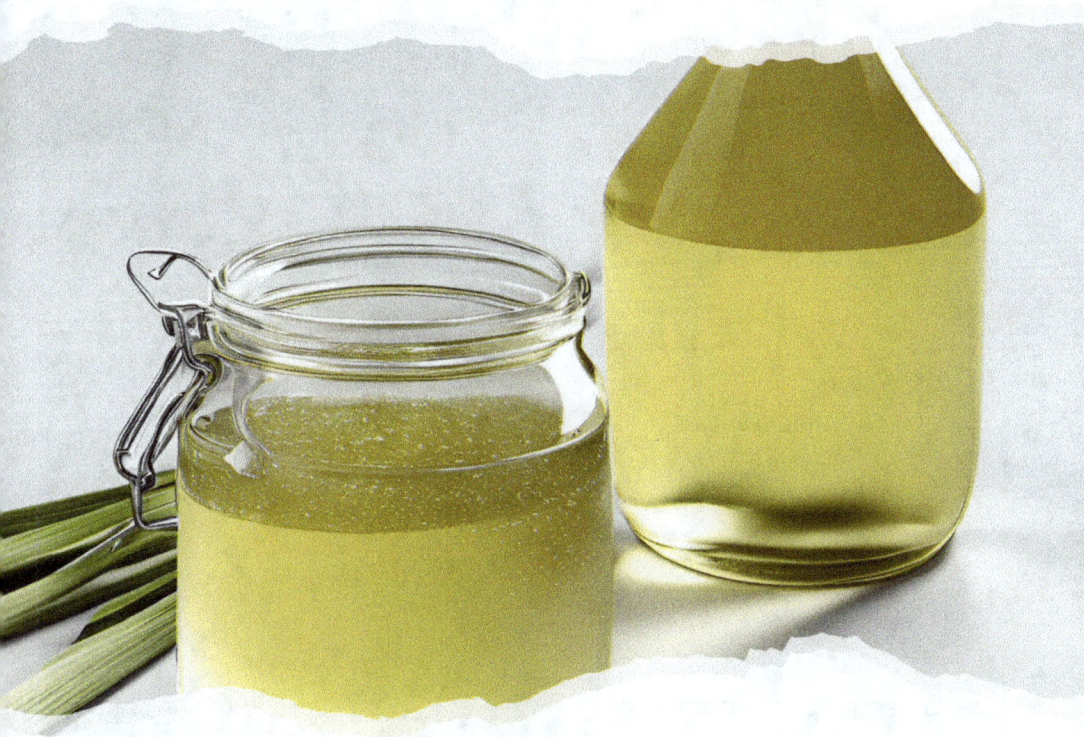

Ingredients

- 1 cup water
- 1 cup granulated sugar
- 2 lemongrass stalks (cut into pieces)

Procedure

1. In a saucepan, combine water, sugar, and chopped lemongrass. Bring to a boil, then reduce the heat and simmer for 10 minutes.
2. Remove from heat and let it steep for an additional 15 minutes.
3. Strain out the lemongrass and let the syrup cool before pouring into a sterilized bottle or jar.
4. Store in the refrigerator for up to 2 weeks.

LEMON SYRUP

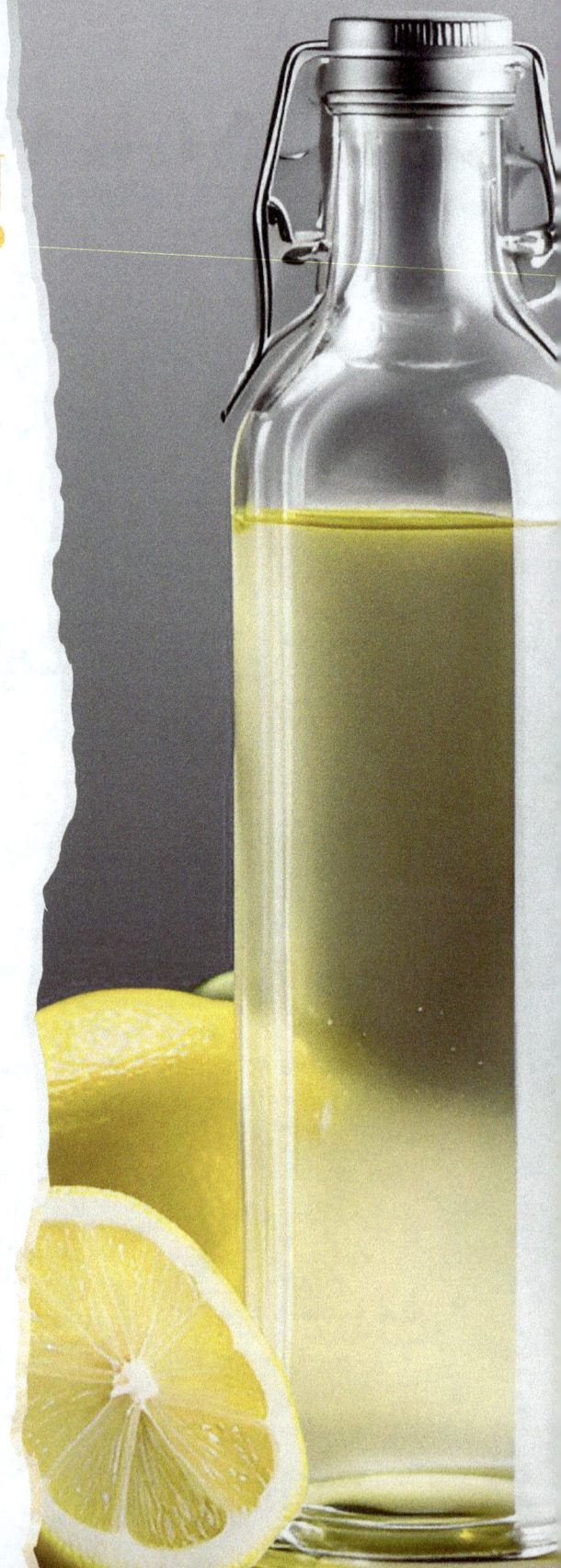

Ingredients

- 1 cup water
- 1 cup granulated sugar
- Zest of 2 lemons

Procedure

1. In a saucepan, combine water, sugar, and lemon zest. Bring to a boil, then reduce the heat and simmer for 5 minutes.
2. Remove from heat and let the syrup cool before pouring into a sterilized bottle or jar.
3. Store in the refrigerator for up to 2 weeks.

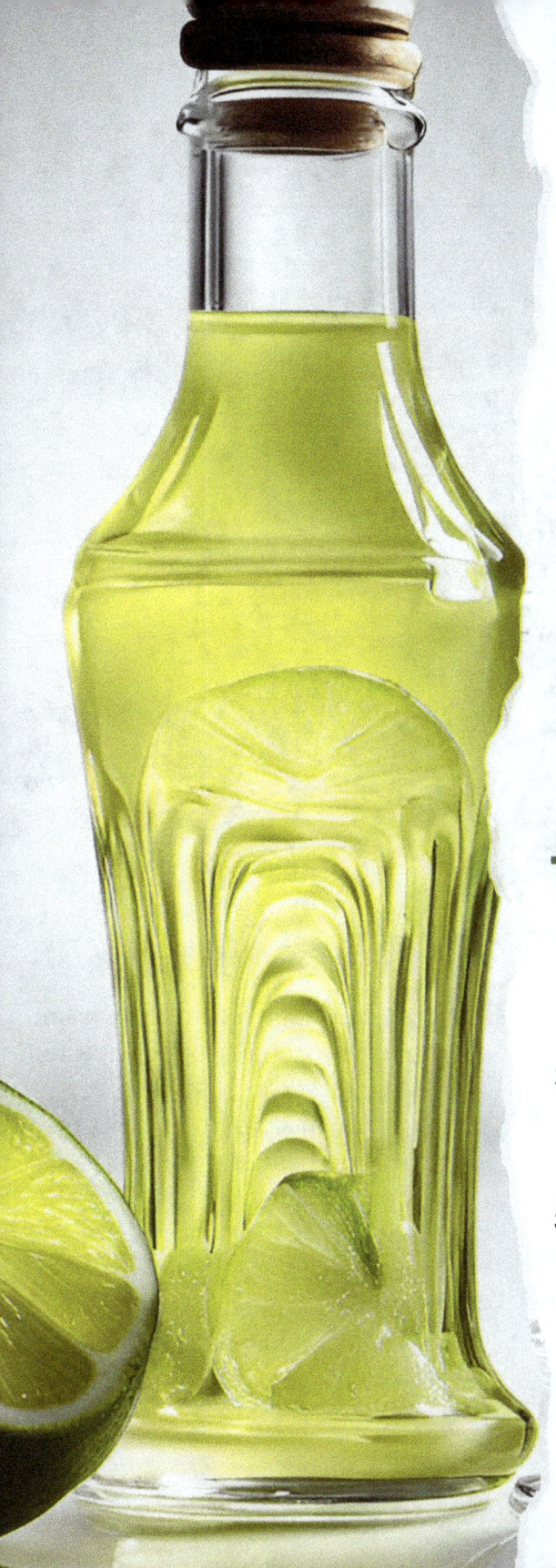

LIME SYRUP

Ingredients

- 1 cup water
- 1 cup granulated sugar
- Zest of 2 limes

Procedure

1. In a saucepan, combine water, sugar, and lime zest. Bring to a boil, then reduce the heat and simmer for 5 minutes.
2. Remove from heat and let the syrup cool before pouring into a sterilized bottle or jar.
3. Store in the refrigerator for up to 2 weeks.

MAPLE PECAN SYRUP

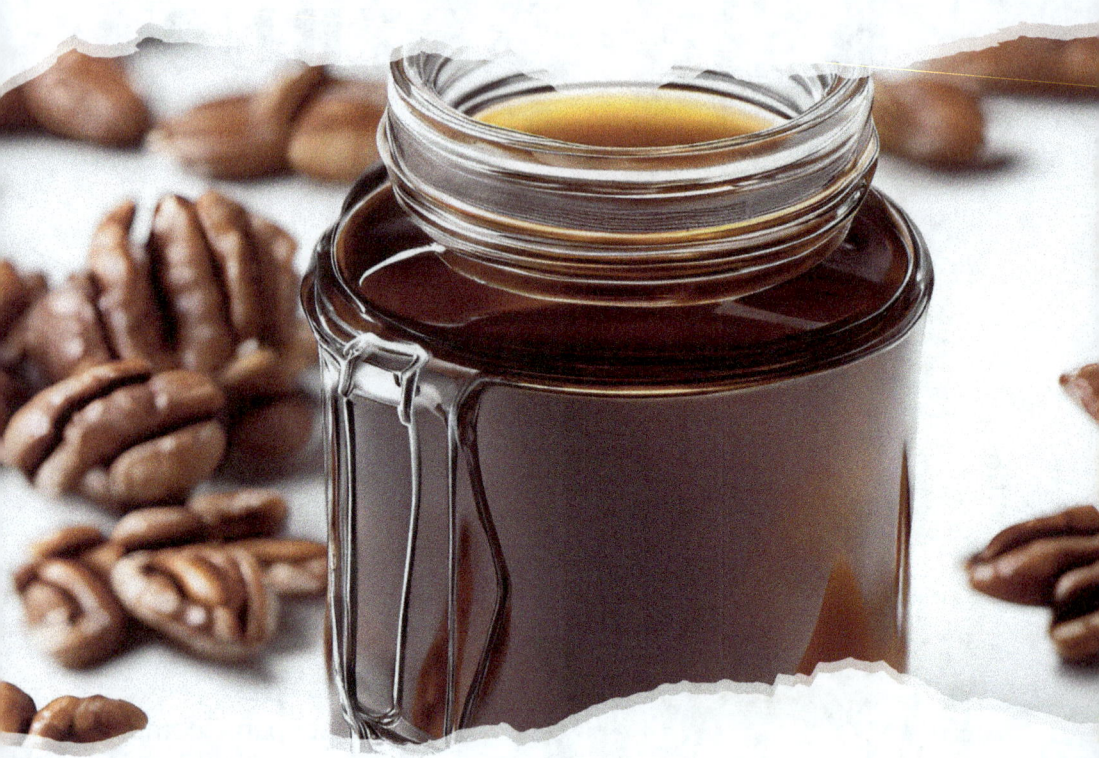

Ingredients

- 1 cup water
- 1/2 cup maple syrup
- 1/2 cup chopped toasted pecans

Procedure

1. In a saucepan, combine water, maple syrup, and chopped toasted pecans.
2. Bring the mixture to a boil, then reduce the heat and simmer for 10 minutes.
3. Remove from heat and let it steep for 15 minutes.
4. Strain out the pecans and pour the syrup into a sterilized bottle or jar.
5. Store in the refrigerator for up to 2 weeks.

ORANGE ZEST SYRUP

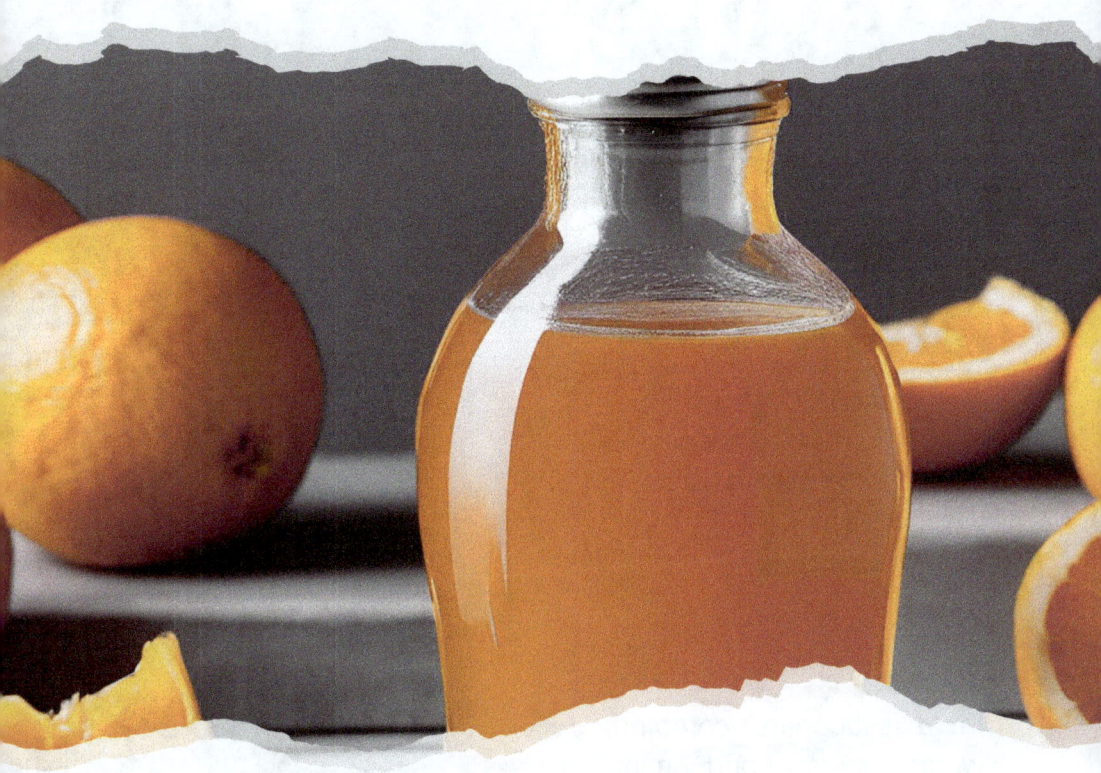

Ingredients

- 1 cup water
- 1 cup granulated sugar
- Zest of 2 oranges thinly peeled orange skin without the white pith attached.

Procedure

1. In a saucepan, combine water, sugar, and orange zest. Bring to a boil, then reduce the heat and simmer for 5 minutes.
2. Remove from heat and let the syrup cool before pouring into a sterilized bottle or jar.
3. Store in the refrigerator for up to 2 weeks.

MINT SYRUP

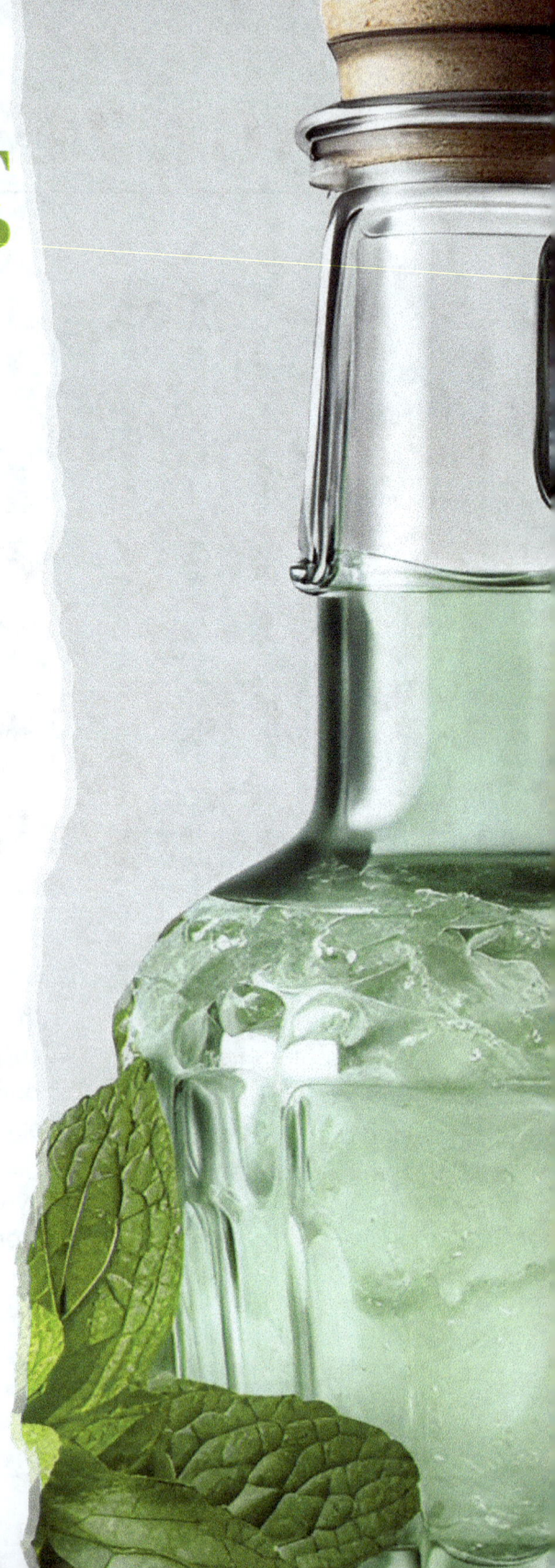

Ingredients

- 1 cup water
- 1 cup granulated sugar
- 1 cup fresh mint leaves

Procedure

1. In a saucepan, combine water, sugar, and mint leaves. Bring to a boil, then reduce the heat and simmer for 5 minutes.
2. Remove from heat and let the syrup steep for 15 minutes.
3. Strain out the mint leaves and let the syrup cool before pouring into a sterilized bottle or jar.
4. Store in the refrigerator for up to 2 weeks.

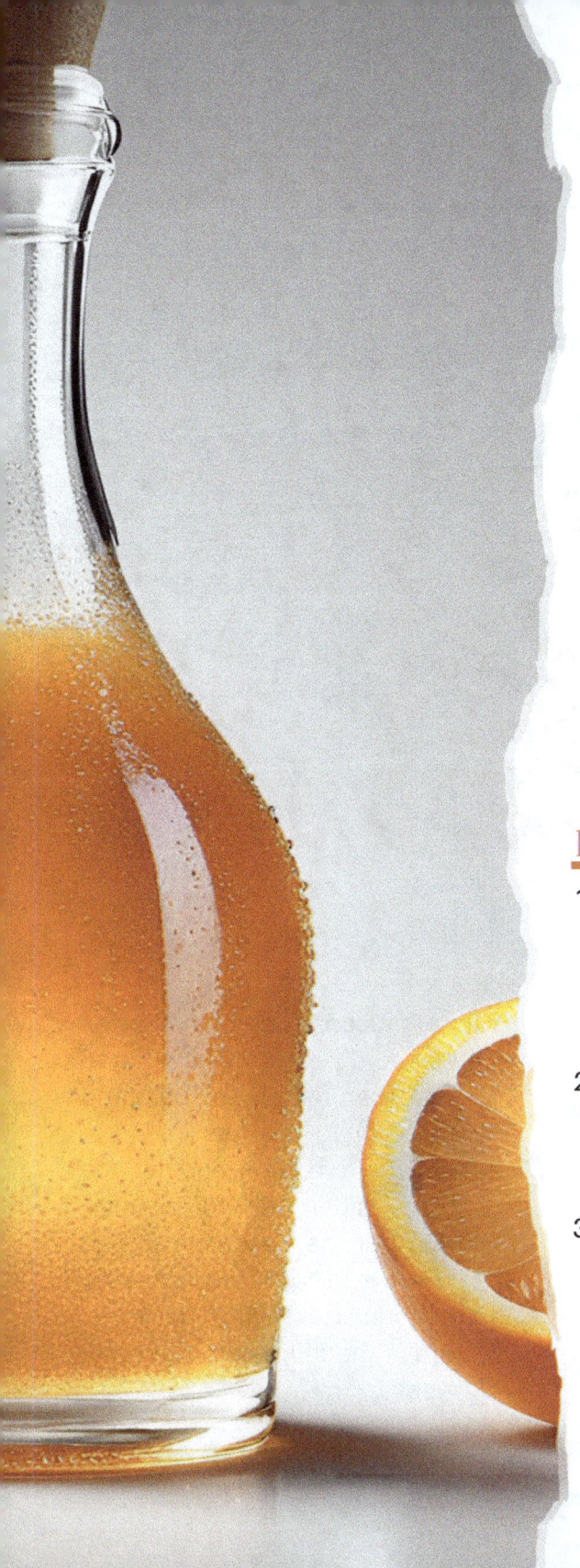

ORANGE SYRUP

Ingredients

- 1/2 cup water
- 1/2 cup orange juice
- 1 cup granulated sugar
- Zest of 1 orange thinly peeled orange skin without the white pith attached.

Procedure

1. In a saucepan, combine water, juice, sugar, and orange zest. Bring to a boil, then reduce the heat and simmer for 5 minutes.
2. Remove from heat and let the syrup cool before pouring into a sterilized bottle or jar.
3. Store in the refrigerator for up to 2 weeks.

PEACH SYRUP

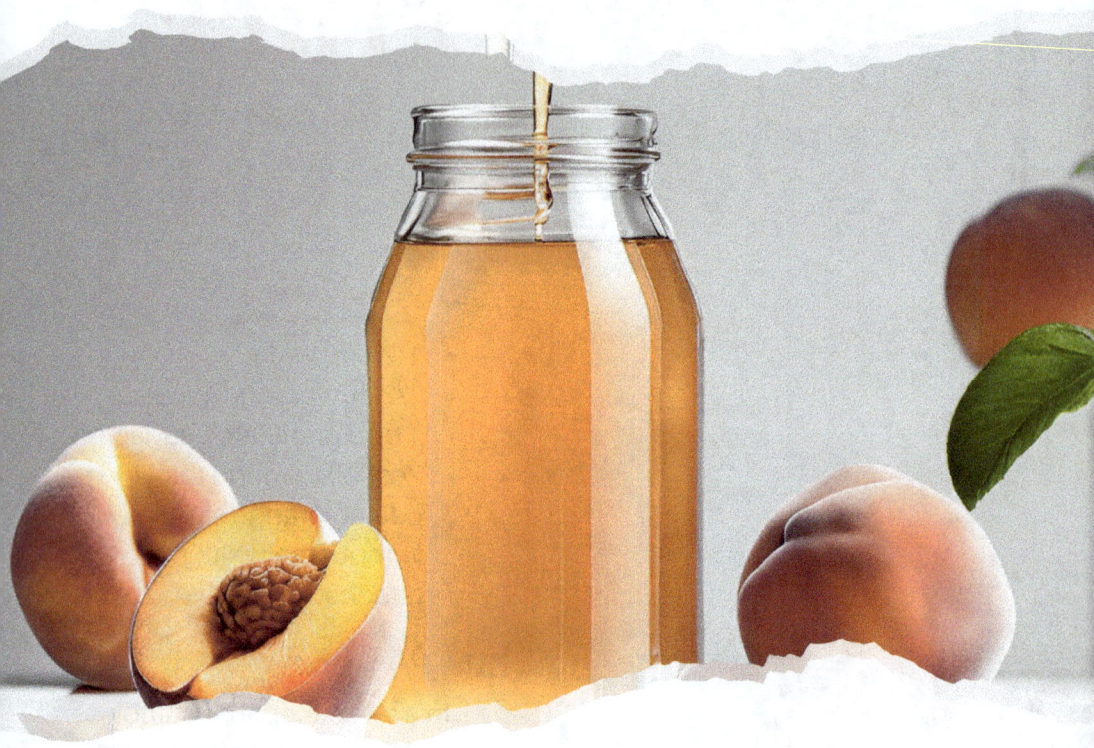

Ingredients

- 1 cup water
- 1 cup granulated sugar
- 1 cup fresh peach slices

Procedure

1. In a saucepan, combine water, sugar, and peach slices. Bring to a boil, then reduce the heat and simmer for 10 minutes.
2. Remove from heat and let the mixture steep for 15 minutes. Strain out the peach slices and let the syrup cool before pouring into a sterilized bottle or jar.
3. Store in the refrigerator for up to 2 weeks.

PUMPKIN SPICE SYRUP

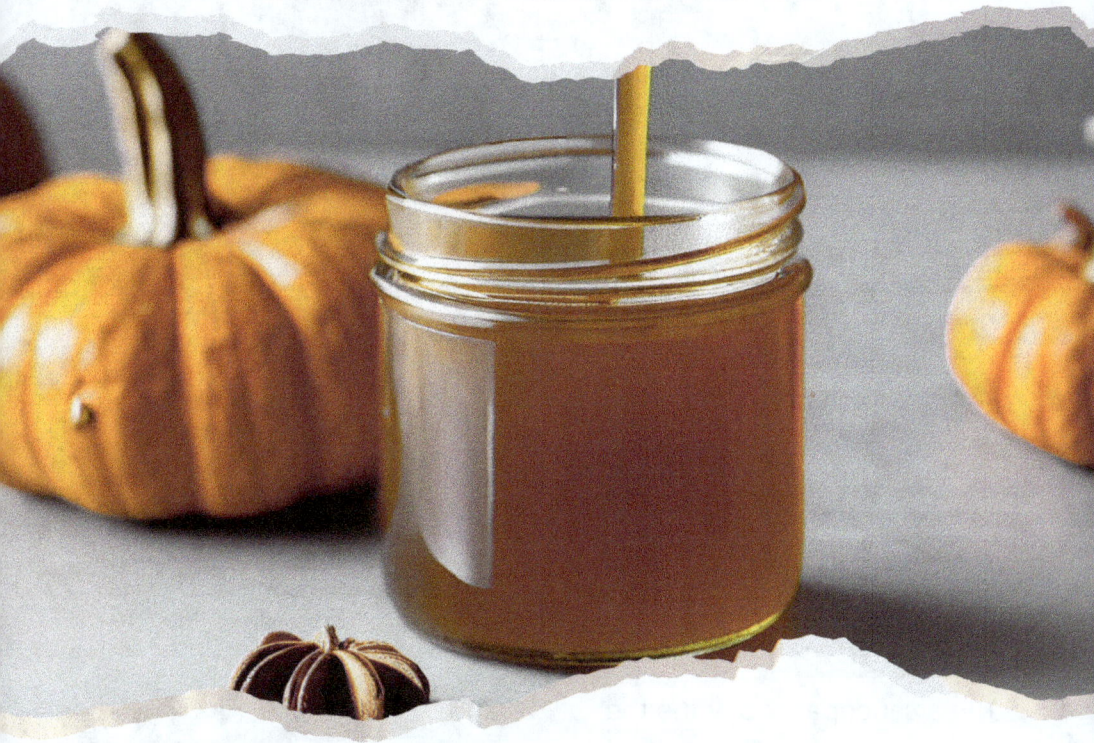

Ingredients

- 1 cup water
- 1 cup granulated sugar
- 2 tablespoons pumpkin puree
- 1/2 teaspoon ground cinnamon
- 1/4 teaspoon ground nutmeg
- 1/4 teaspoon ground cloves

Procedure

1. In a saucepan, combine the water, sugar, pumpkin puree, and spices. Bring the mixture to a boil, then reduce the heat and simmer for 5 minutes.
2. Remove from heat and let the syrup cool slightly.
3. Strain through a fine mesh sieve to remove any solids, then pour the syrup into a sterilized bottle or jar.
4. Store in the refrigerator for up to 1 week.

PEPPERMINT SYRUP

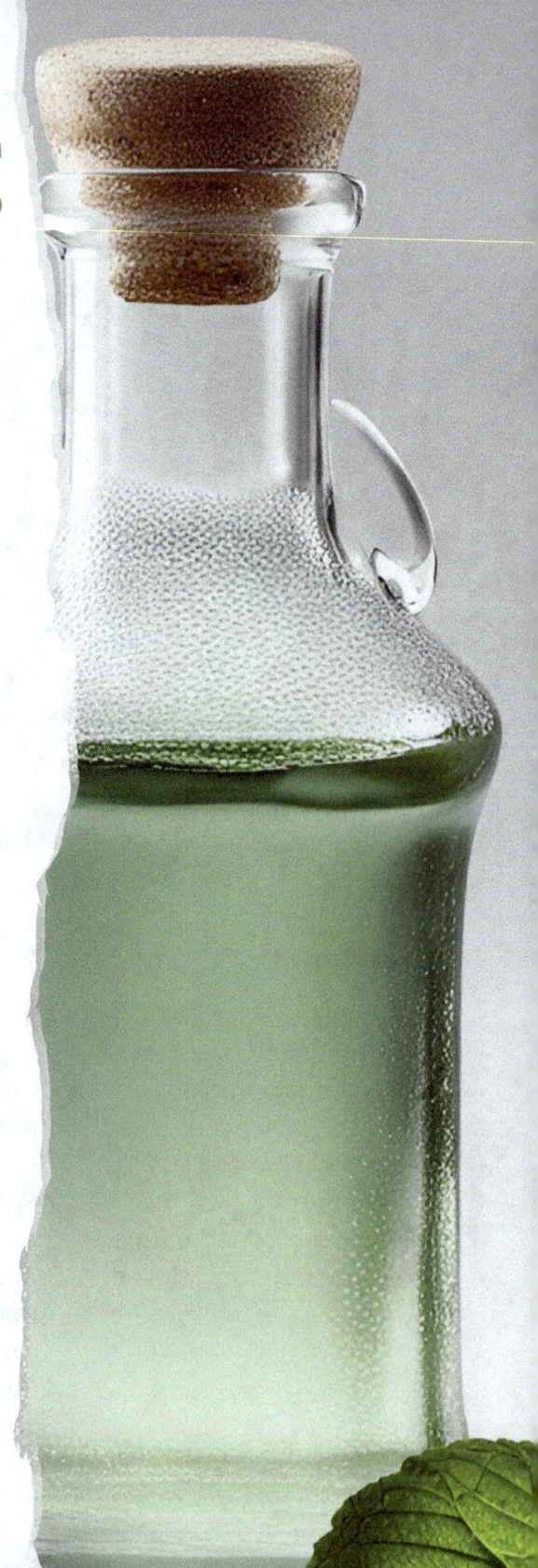

Ingredients

- 1 cup water
- 1 cup granulated sugar
- 1 cup fresh peppermint leaves

Note: Peppermint has a different, stronger flavor than mint. However mint syrup and peppermint syrup can be used interchangeably.

Procedure

1. In a saucepan, combine the water, sugar, and peppermint leaves.
2. Bring the mixture to a boil, then reduce the heat and simmer for 5 minutes.
3. Remove from heat and let the syrup steep for 15 minutes to infuse the peppermint flavor.
4. Strain out the leaves and pour the syrup into a sterilized bottle or jar.
5. Store in the refrigerator for up to 2 weeks.

ROSE SYRUP

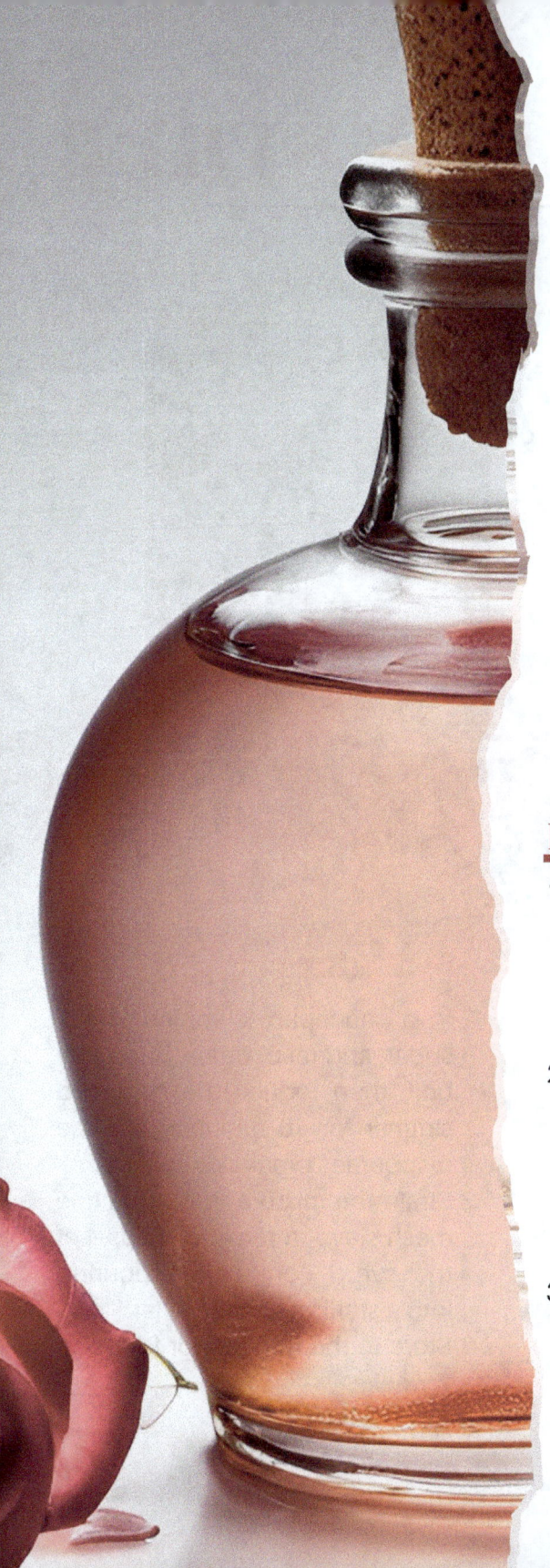

Ingredients

- 1 cup water
- 1 cup granulated sugar
- 1/2 cup fresh or 1/2 cup dried rose petals (organic and food-grade)

Procedure

1. In a saucepan, combine water, sugar, and rose petals. Bring to a boil, then reduce the heat and simmer for 5 minutes.
2. Remove from heat and let the syrup steep for 15 minutes. Strain out the rose petals and let the syrup cool before pouring into a sterilized bottle or jar.
3. Store in the refrigerator for up to 2 weeks.

RASPBERRY SYRUP

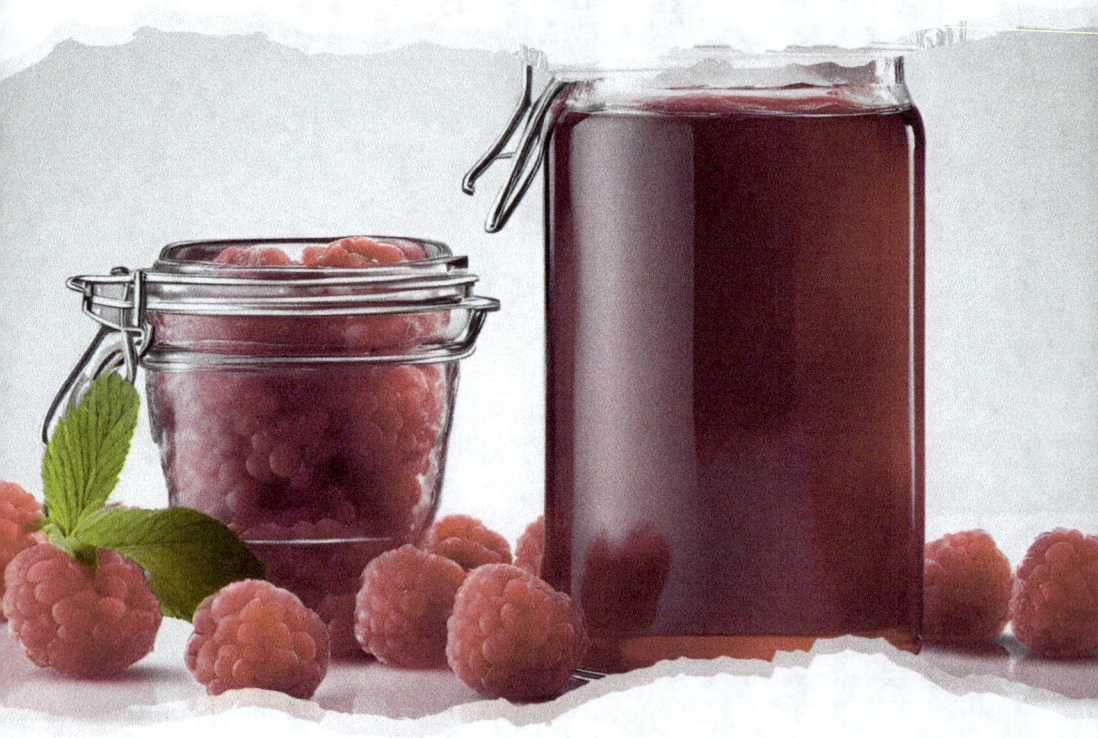

Ingredients

- 1 cup water
- 1 cup granulated sugar
- 1 cup fresh raspberries

Procedure

1. In a saucepan, combine water, sugar, and raspberries. Bring to a boil, then reduce the heat and simmer for 10 minutes until the raspberries break down.
2. Strain the mixture through a fine mesh sieve to remove seeds. Let the syrup cool before pouring into a sterilized bottle or jar.
3. Store in the refrigerator for up to 2 weeks.

SPICED CLOVE SYRUP

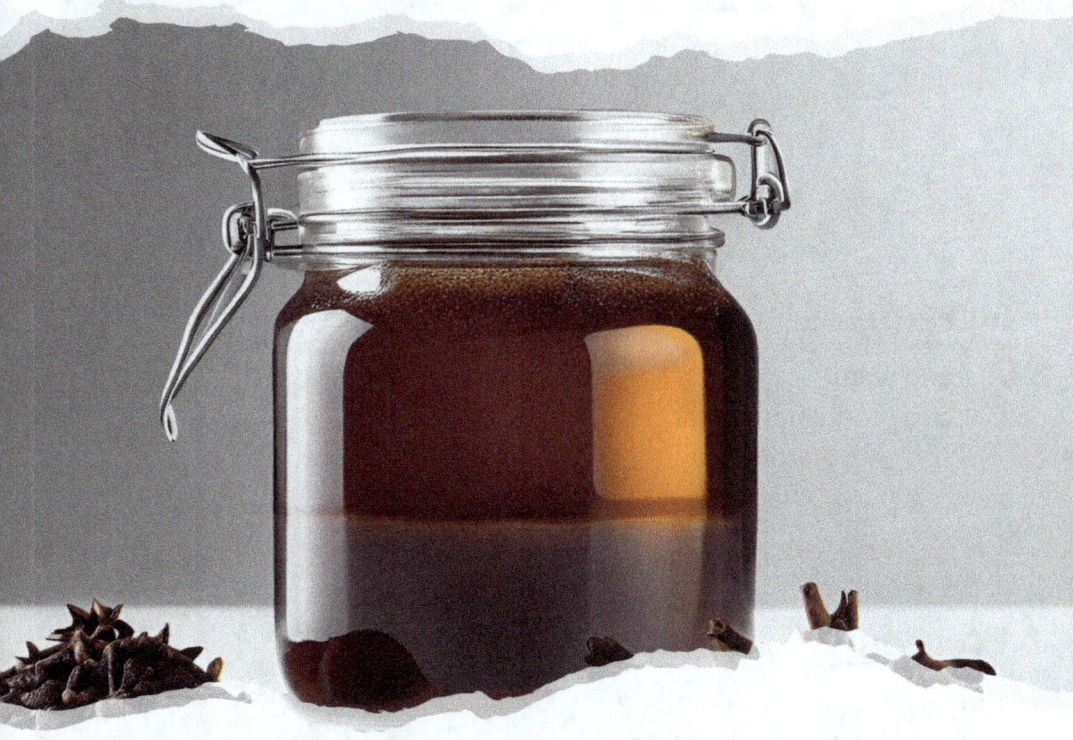

Ingredients
- 1 cup water
- 1 cup granulated sugar
- 1 tablespoon whole cloves

Procedure
1. In a saucepan, combine water, sugar, and cloves. Bring to a boil, then reduce the heat and simmer for 5 minutes.
2. Remove from heat and let the syrup steep for 15 minutes.
3. Strain out the cloves and let the syrup cool before pouring into a sterilized bottle or jar.
4. Store in the refrigerator for up to 2 weeks.

ROSEMARY SYRUP

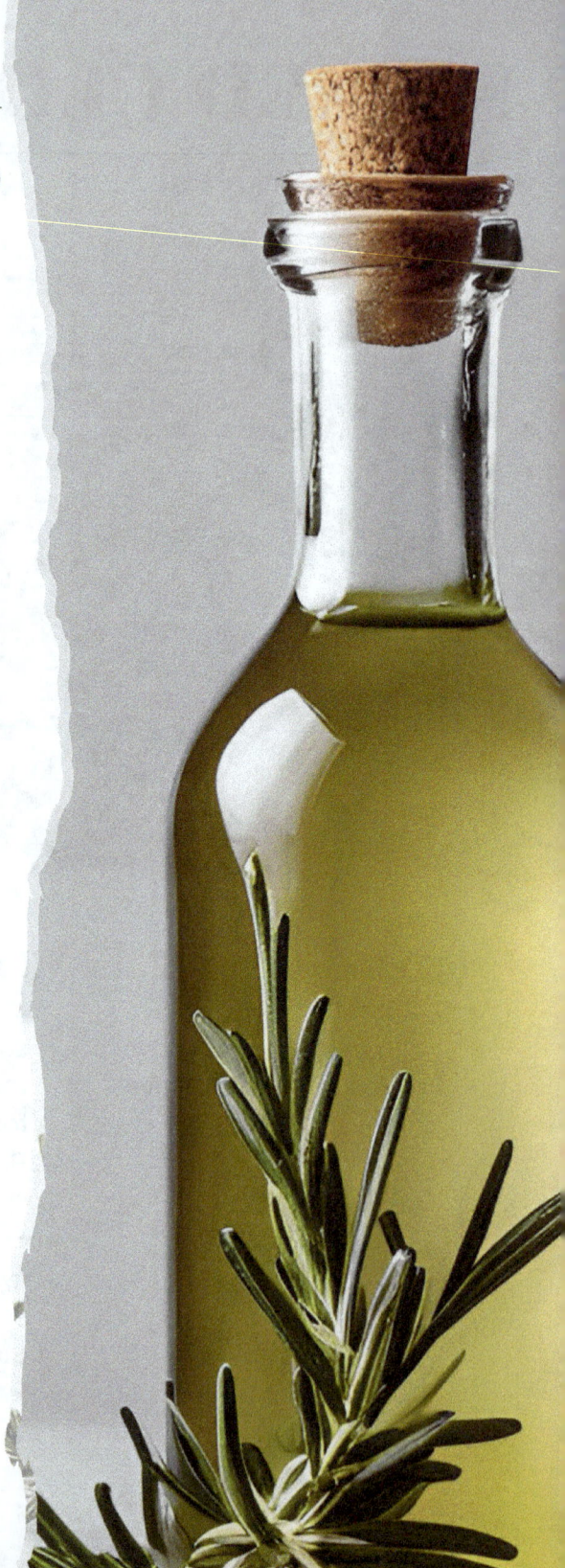

Ingredients

- 1 cup water
- 1 cup granulated sugar
- 3 sprigs fresh rosemary

Procedure

1. In a saucepan, combine water, sugar, and rosemary sprigs. Bring to a boil, then reduce the heat and simmer for 5 minutes.
2. Remove from heat and let the syrup steep for 15 minutes.
3. Strain out the rosemary sprigs and let the infusion cool before pouring into a sterilized bottle or jar.
4. Store in the refrigerator for up to 2 weeks.

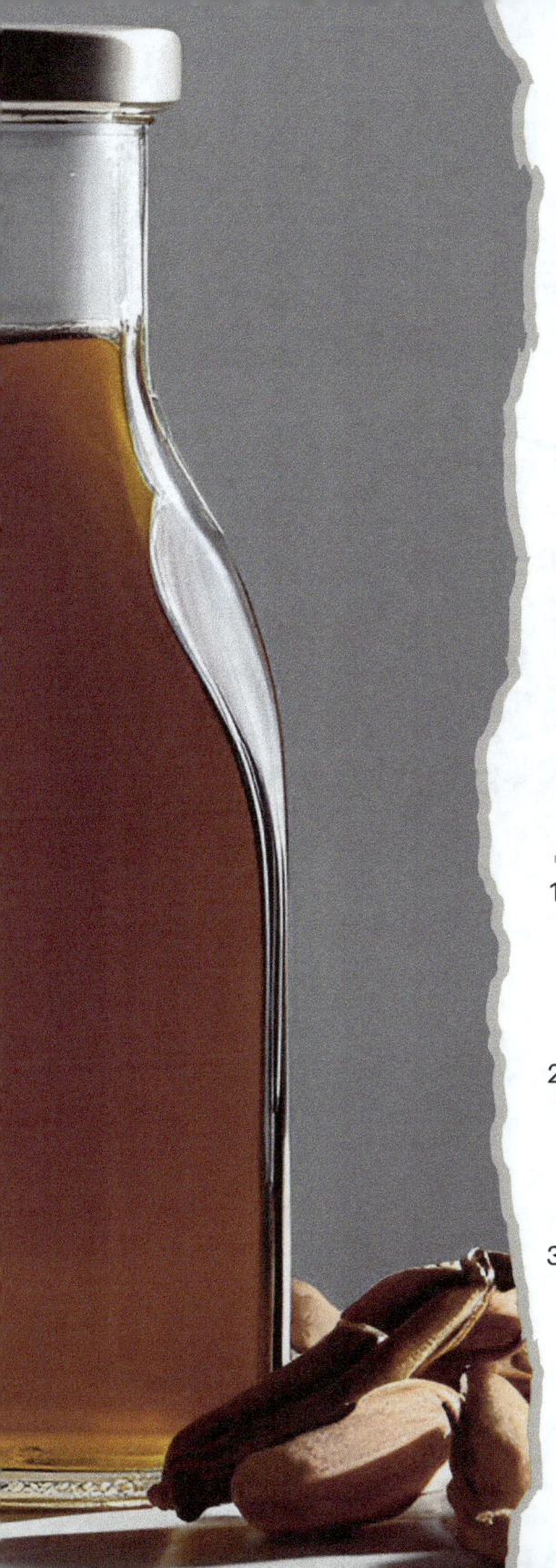

TAMARIND SYRUP

Ingredients

- 1 cup water
- 1 cup granulated sugar
- 1 cup tamarind pulp (or 1/2 cup tamarind paste)

Procedure

1. In a saucepan, combine the tamarind pulp, water, and sugar. Bring to a boil, then reduce the heat and simmer for 10 minutes.
2. Strain the mixture through a fine mesh sieve to remove seeds and pulp. Let the syrup cool before pouring into a sterilized bottle or jar.
3. Store in the refrigerator for up to 2 weeks.

VANILLA BEAN SYRUP

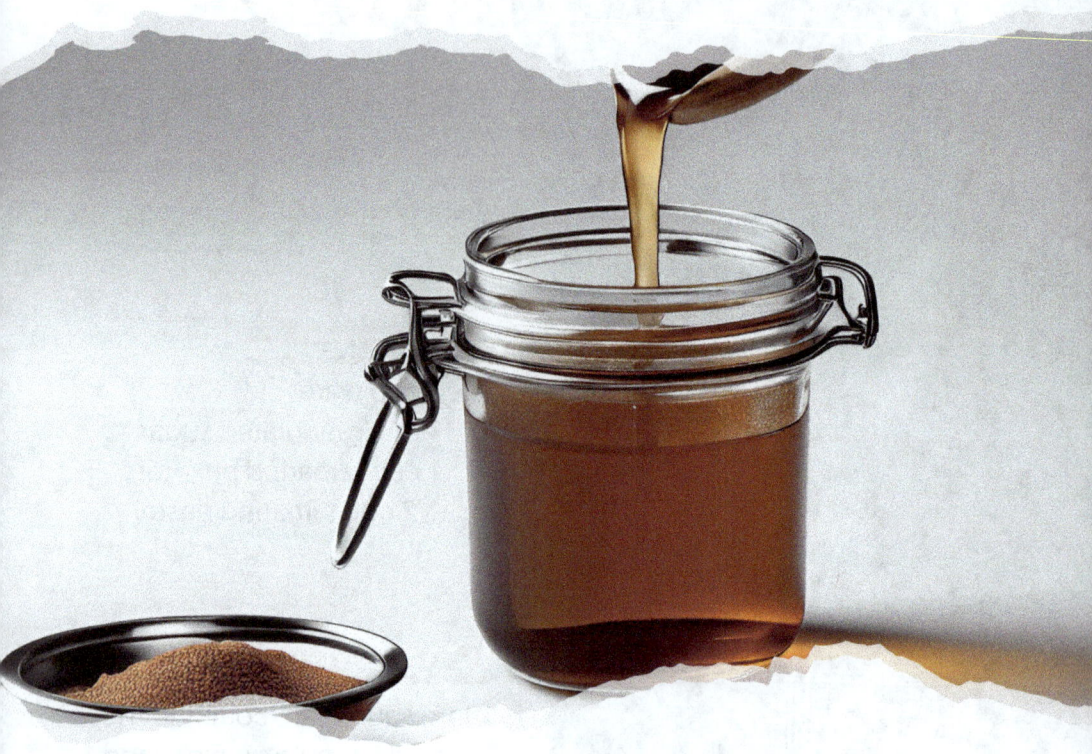

Ingredients

- 1 cup water
- 1 cup granulated sugar
- 1 vanilla bean, split
- Option: add 1/2 teaspoon freshly grated nutmeg to the saucepan in step 1 to make a Vanilla Nutmeg Syrup.

Procedure

1. In a saucepan, combine water, sugar, and the split vanilla bean. Bring to a boil, then reduce the heat and simmer for 5 minutes.
2. Remove from heat and let the syrup steep for 15 minutes.
3. Remove the vanilla bean and let the syrup cool before pouring into a sterilized bottle or jar.
4. Store in the refrigerator for up to 2 weeks.

VIOLET SYRUP

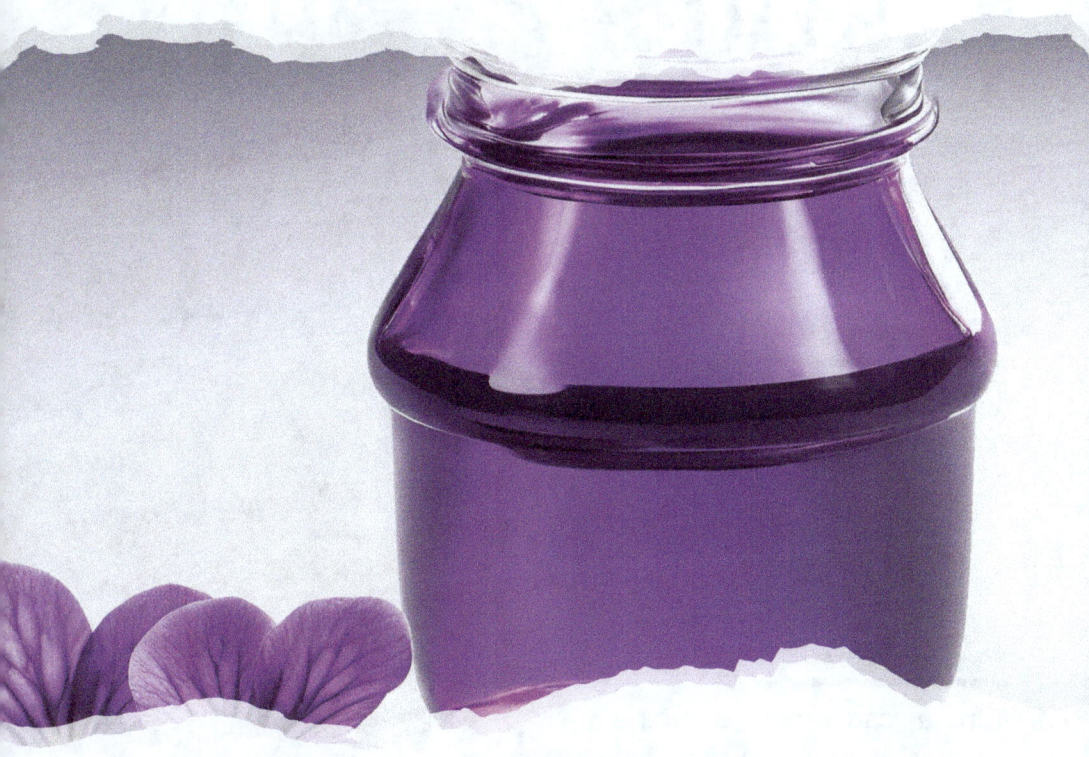

Ingredients

- 1 cup water
- 1 cup granulated sugar
- 1/2 cup fresh violet flowers (or 1 tablespoon dried, food-grade violet flowers)

Procedure

1. In a saucepan, combine water, sugar, and violet flowers. Bring to a boil, then reduce the heat and simmer for 5 minutes.
2. Remove from heat and let the syrup steep for 15 minutes.
3. Strain out the violet flowers and let the syrup cool before pouring into a sterilized bottle or jar.
4. Store in the refrigerator for up to 2 weeks.

THYME SYRUP

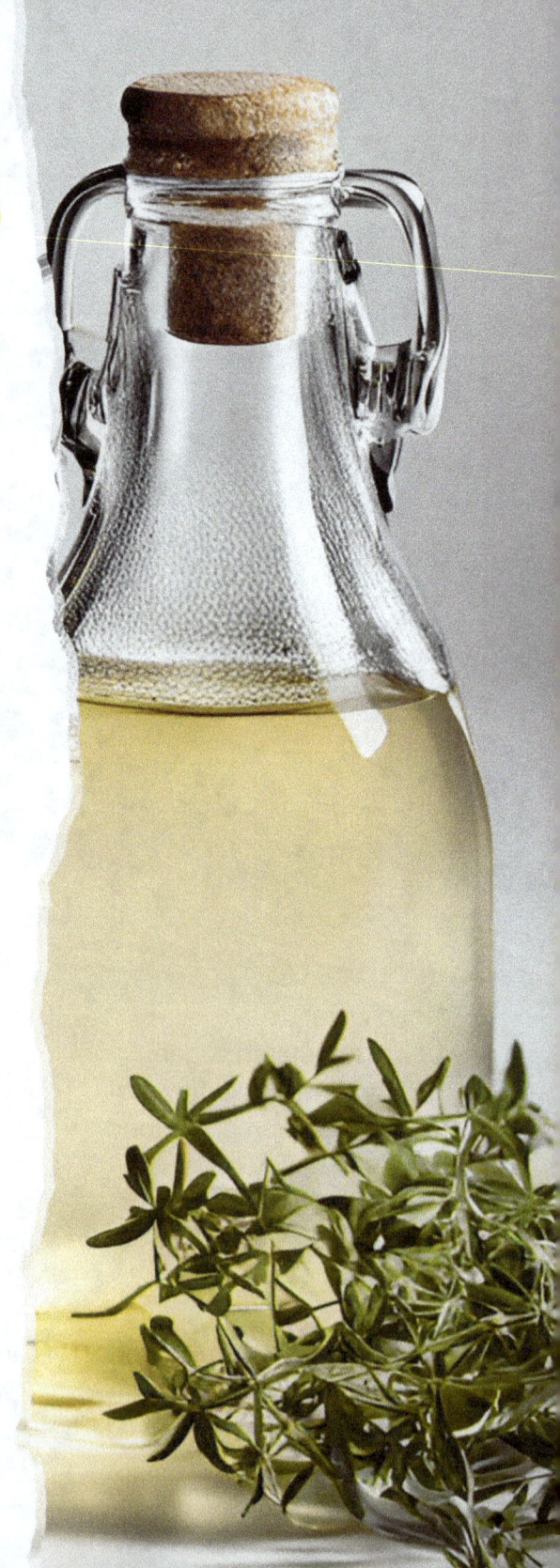

Ingredients

- 1 cup water
- 1 cup granulated sugar
- 5 sprigs fresh thyme

Procedure

1. In a saucepan, combine water, sugar, and thyme sprigs. Bring to a boil, then reduce the heat and simmer for 5 minutes.
2. Remove from heat and let the mixture steep for 15 minutes.
3. Strain out the thyme and let the infusion cool before pouring into a sterilized bottle or jar.
4. Store in the refrigerator for up to 2 weeks.

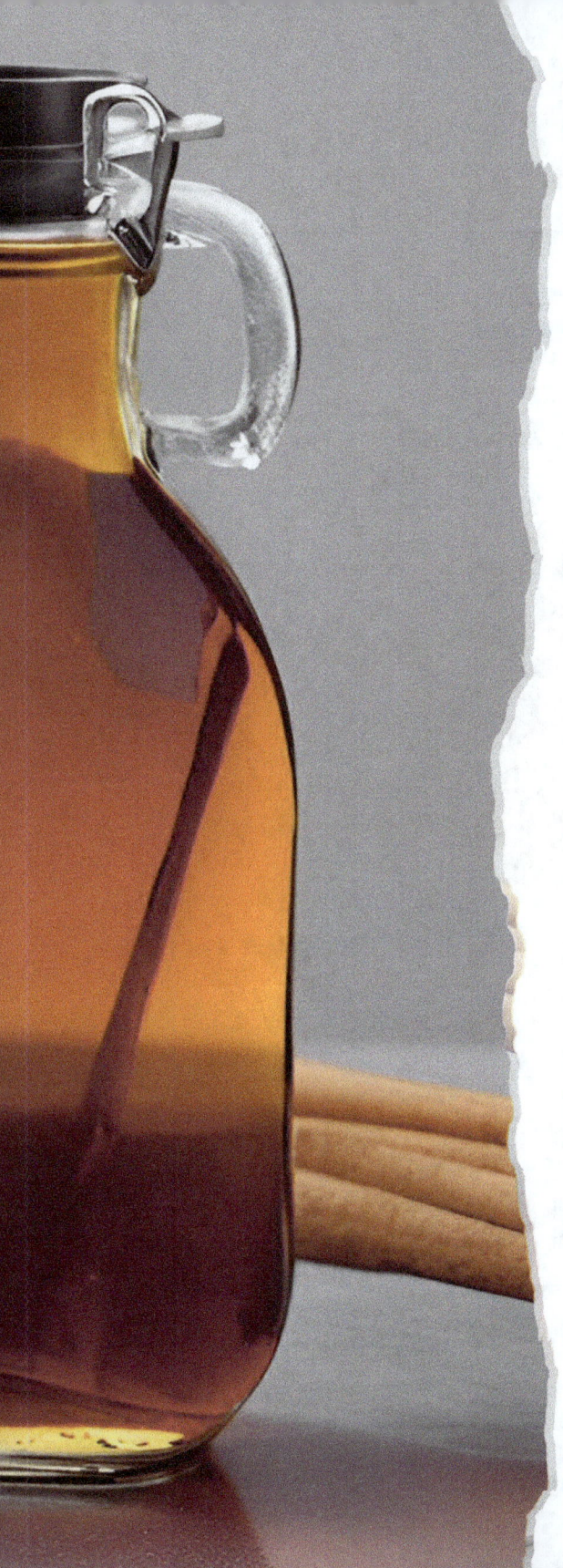

SPICED SYRUP

Ingredients

- 1 cup water
- 1 cup coconut sugar (or maple syrup)
- 1 cinnamon stick
- 3 whole cloves
- 2 cardamom pods (crushed)
- 1 piece of fresh ginger (1-inch slice)
- Optional: 1/2 vanilla bean (or 1 tsp vanilla extract)

Procedure

1. Combine all ingredients in a saucepan and bring to a boil.
2. Reduce heat to low and simmer for 10-15 minutes.
3. Strain into a glass jar and store in the fridge for up to 2 weeks.

HONEY-GINGER SYRUP

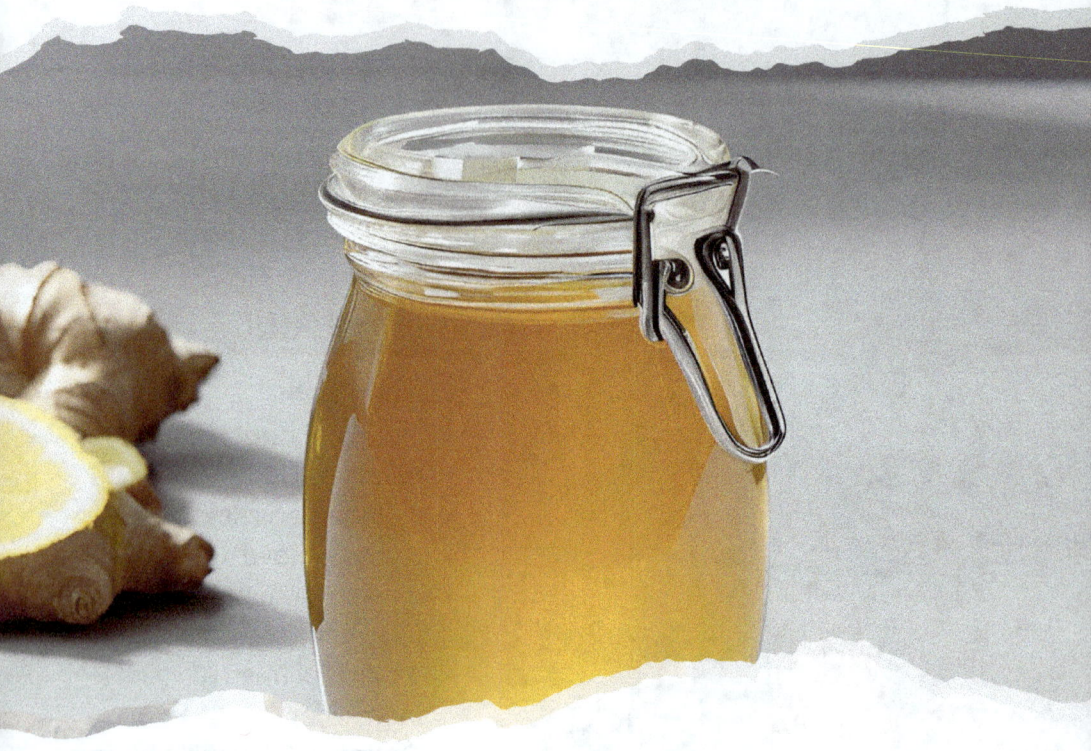

Ingredients

- 1 cup honey (or 1/2 cup honey + 1/2 cup water for a thinner syrup)
- 1-inch fresh ginger, peeled and sliced
- 1 cinnamon stick (optional)
- 1 tsp lemon juice (optional, for a citrus twist)

Procedure

1. Combine honey, water (if using), ginger, and cinnamon in a small saucepan.
2. Warm over low heat (do not boil) for 10-15 minutes.
3. Remove from heat and add the lemon juice, if using.
4. Strain the syrup into a jar or bottle.
5. Store in the refrigerator for up to 2 weeks.

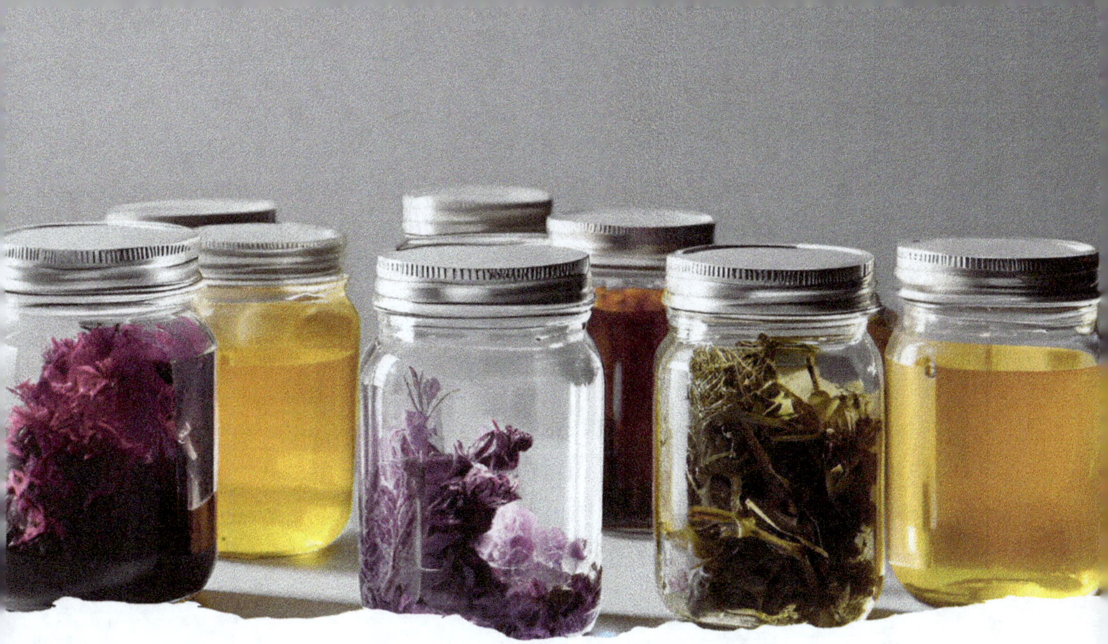

INFUSIONS

Delicate and aromatic, these infusions bring the essence of fresh herbs, fragrant teas, and edible flowers to your mocktails, adding layers of complexity and elegance.

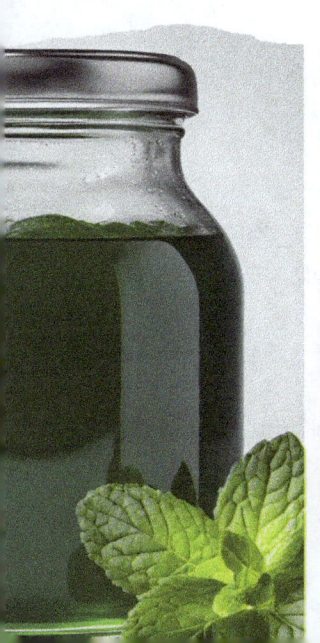
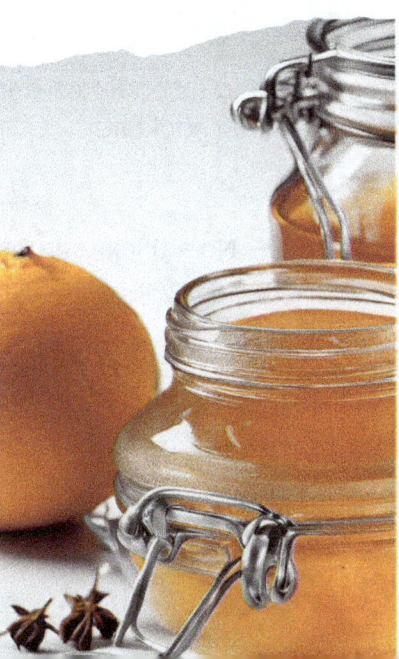
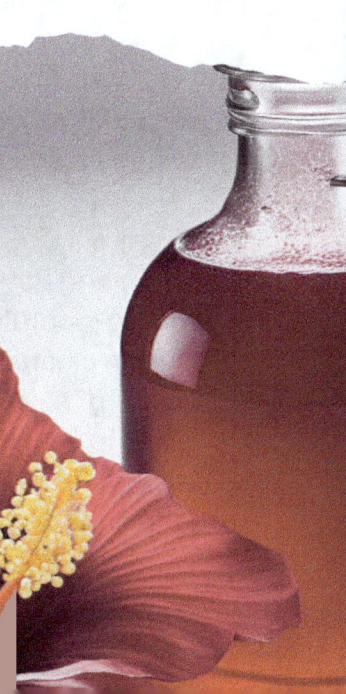

What is an infusion?

Although the terms 'syrup' and 'infusions' are sometimes used interchangeably, in this book we are separating them based on whether they are simple-syrup-based (with sugar) or made without sugar.

An infusion is the process of steeping or soaking ingredients in a liquid to extract their flavor. In mocktails, this usually involves infusing:
- **Water:** for flavored ice cubes or tea-based mocktails
- **Syrups:** to add depth and natural complexity
- **Juices:** enhancing citrus or fruit-based drinks
- **Milk or nut milks such as Coconut Milk:** for creamy, dessert-style mocktail

Infusions: Unlocking Depth & Complexity in Mocktails
Mocktails are more than just fruit juice and soda—they're an artful balance of flavors, aromas, and textures. One of the best ways to elevate your mocktail game is by using infusions, which add depth, complexity, and sophistication to your drinks without alcohol.

Infusions allow you to extract subtle, layered flavors from herbs, spices, fruits, teas, and botanicals. Whether you want a spicy kick of ginger, the floral sweetness of lavender, or the earthy warmth of chai, infusions help transform simple ingredients into something extraordinary.

Why Use Infusions in Mocktails?
Infusions bring a gourmet touch to alcohol-free drinks, making them feel just as elegant and refined as a craft cocktail.

Properties of infusions
- **Enhancing flavor naturally** – No artificial syrups or extracts needed.
- **Adding complexity** – A rosemary-infused syrup or a vanilla bean infusion creates layers of taste.
- **Creating a signature drink** – Infusions allow you to personalize flavors to your liking.
- **Giving a sophisticated, "grown-up" feel** – Perfect for alcohol-free gatherings or mindful drinking.

How to Make a Simple Infusion
The method depends on your ingredients, but here's a basic approach:
- Choose Your Base Liquid – Water, syrup, juice, tea, or milk.
- Select Your Infusion Ingredient – Fresh herbs, dried spices, citrus peels, fruit, or floral elements.
- Gently Heat (If Needed) – Some infusions work best when gently heated (like vanilla in syrup or cinnamon in milk).
- Let It Steep – From 30 minutes to 24 hours, depending on the intensity you want.
- Strain & Store – Use a fine mesh strainer or cheesecloth for a smooth, clean result.

Infusion Ideas for Mocktails
In addition to the recipes outlined in this book, here are some more ideas:

Herbal Infusions:
- Basil in strawberry syrup
- Rosemary in honey syrup
- Mint in lime juice

Citrus & Fruit Infusions:
- Lemon peel in coconut water
- Cherries in black tea
- Passionfruit in sparkling water

Spice & Floral Infusions:
- Cinnamon in apple juice
- Cardamom in vanilla syrup
- Lavender in lemonade

Using Infusions in Mocktails
- Swap for Regular Ingredients – Use an infused syrup instead of plain sugar syrup.
- Build Layered Mocktails – Pair herbal, fruity, and spiced infusions for unique creations.
- Make Flavored Ice Cubes – Freeze infused water for a slow-releasing burst of flavor.
- Use in Desserts & Coffees – Many infusions work beyond mocktails, adding elegance to other treats.

With infusions, you're no longer just making a drink—you're crafting an experience. Whether you go for a soothing chamomile honey syrup, a zesty ginger-lime infusion, or a smoky cinnamon-clove blend, these techniques will transform your mocktails into something truly special.

Now, let's dive into some delicious infusion recipes to get started!

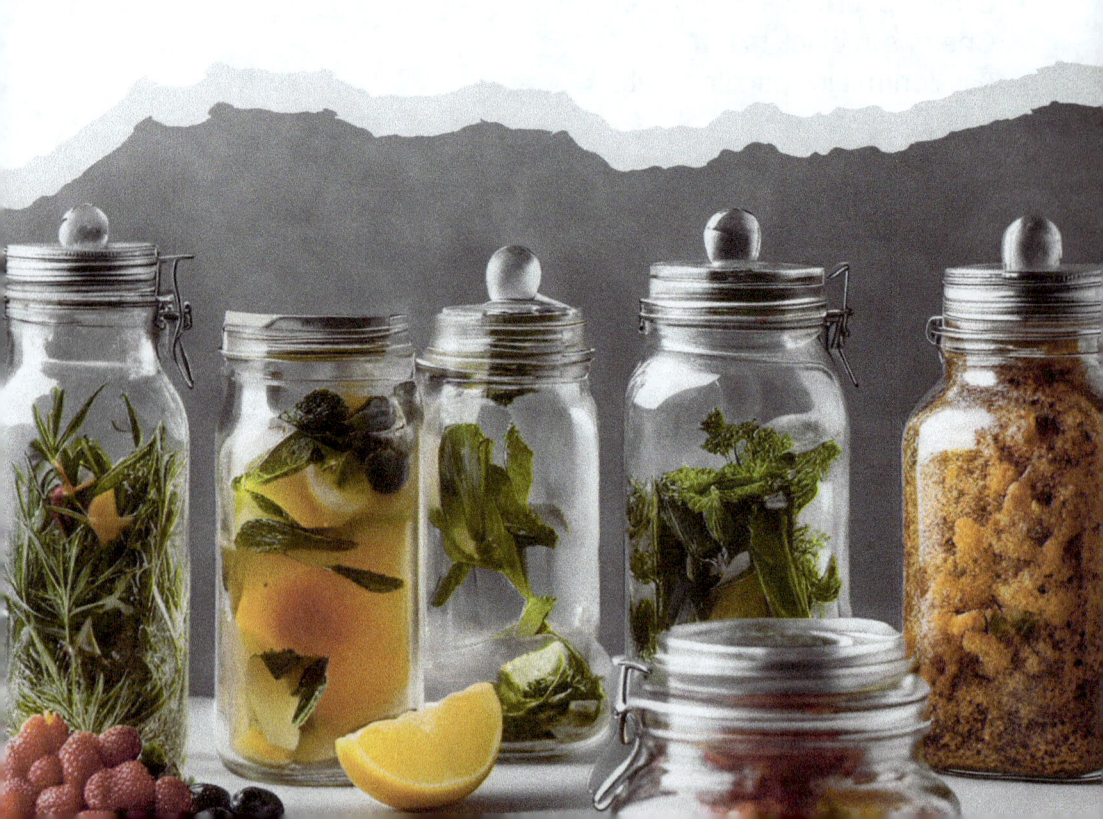

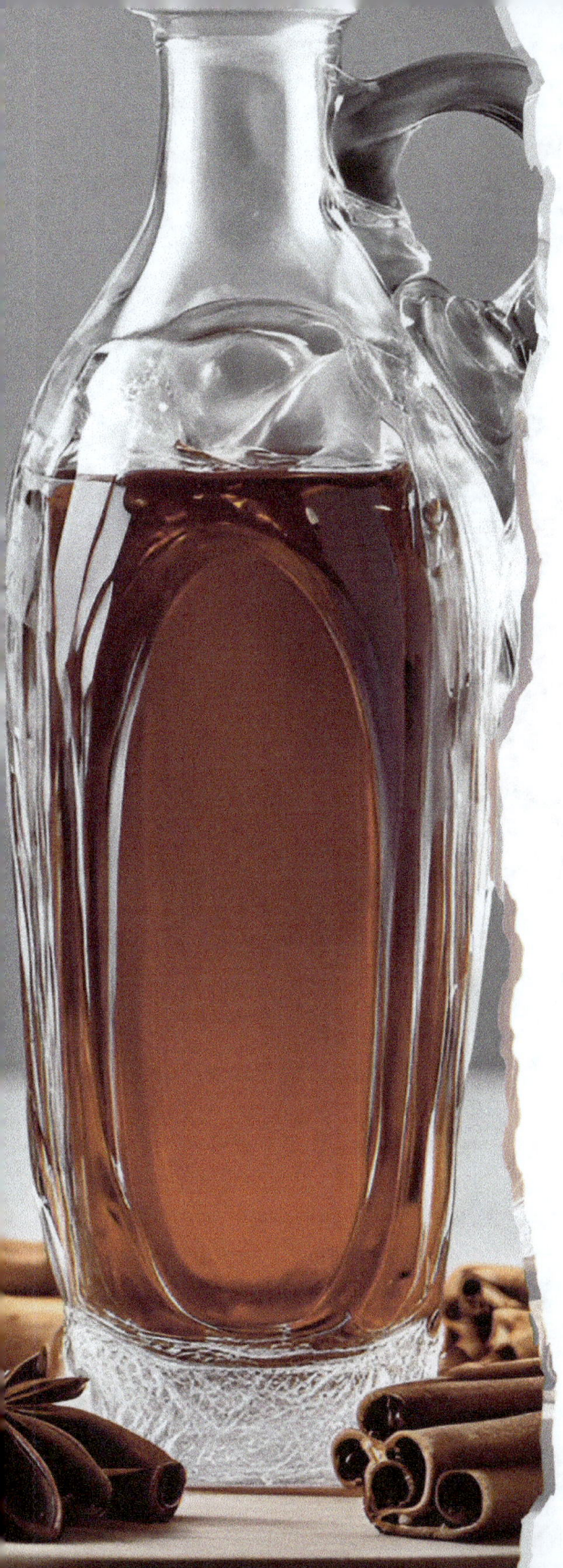

CINNAMON INFUSION

Ingredients

- 1 cup water
- 2 cinnamon sticks

Procedure

1. In a saucepan, bring the water and cinnamon sticks to a boil. Reduce the heat and simmer for 5 minutes.
2. Remove from heat and let it steep for an additional 15 minutes.
3. Strain out the cinnamon sticks and let the infusion cool before pouring into a sterilized bottle or jar.
4. Store in the refrigerator.

CLOVE AND ORANGE

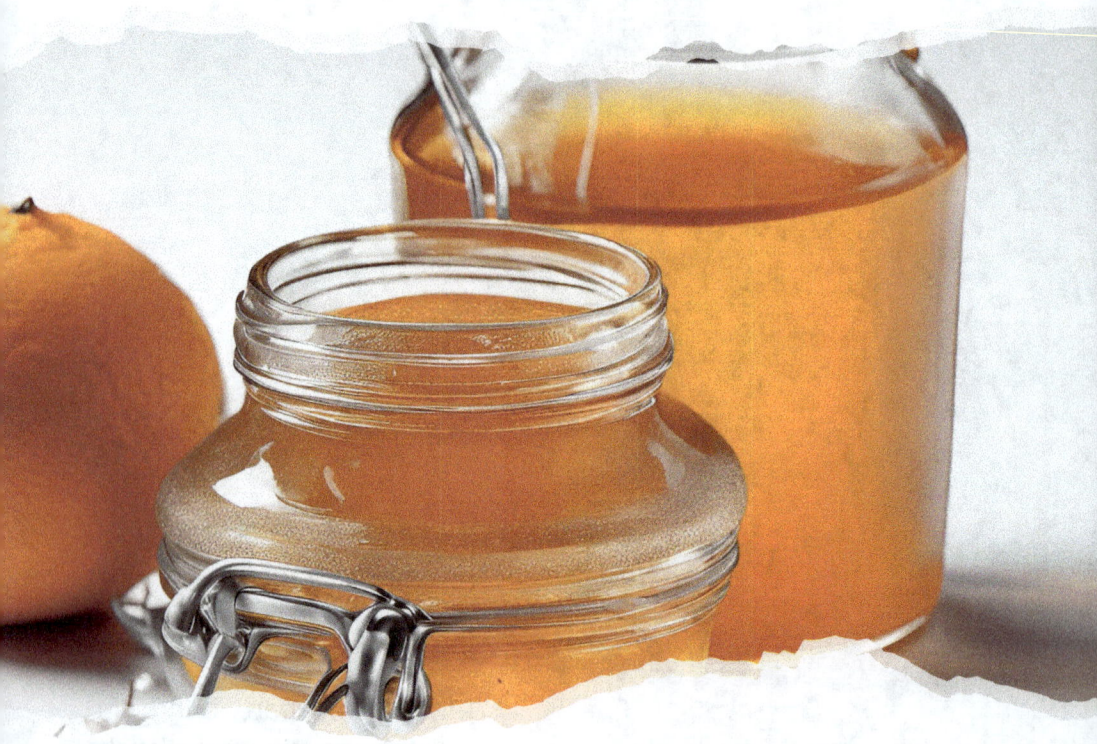

Ingredients

- 1 cup water
- 1 cup granulated sugar
- Zest of 1 orange
- 1 tablespoon whole cloves

Procedure

1. In a saucepan, combine water, orange zest, and cloves.
2. Bring the mixture to a boil, then reduce the heat and simmer for 5 minutes.
3. Remove from heat and let the infusion steep for 15 minutes.
4. Strain out the orange zest and cloves, then pour the infusion into a sterilized bottle or jar.
5. Store in the refrigerator for up to 2 weeks.

MINT INFUSION

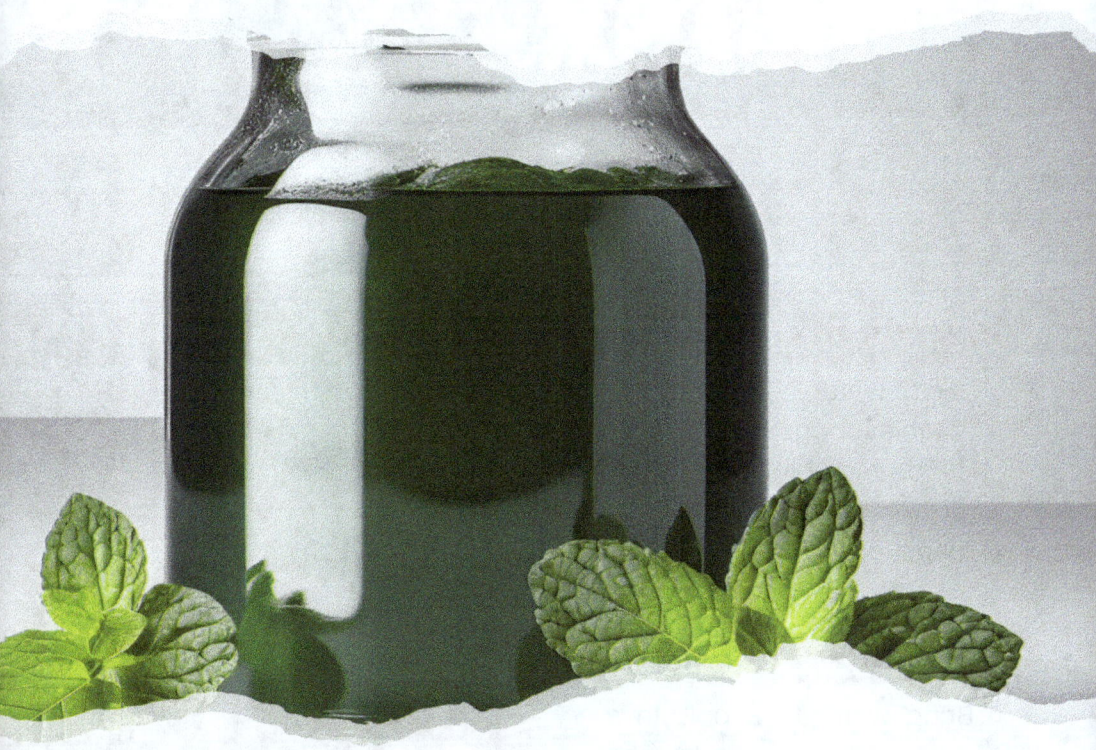

Ingredients

- 1 cup water
- 1 cup fresh mint leaves

Procedure

1. In a saucepan, bring the water to a boil. Add the mint leaves and reduce the heat to a simmer for 5 minutes.
2. Remove from heat and let the infusion steep for 10 minutes. Strain out the mint leaves and let the infusion cool before pouring into a sterilized bottle or jar.
3. Store in the refrigerator.

HIBISCUS TEA

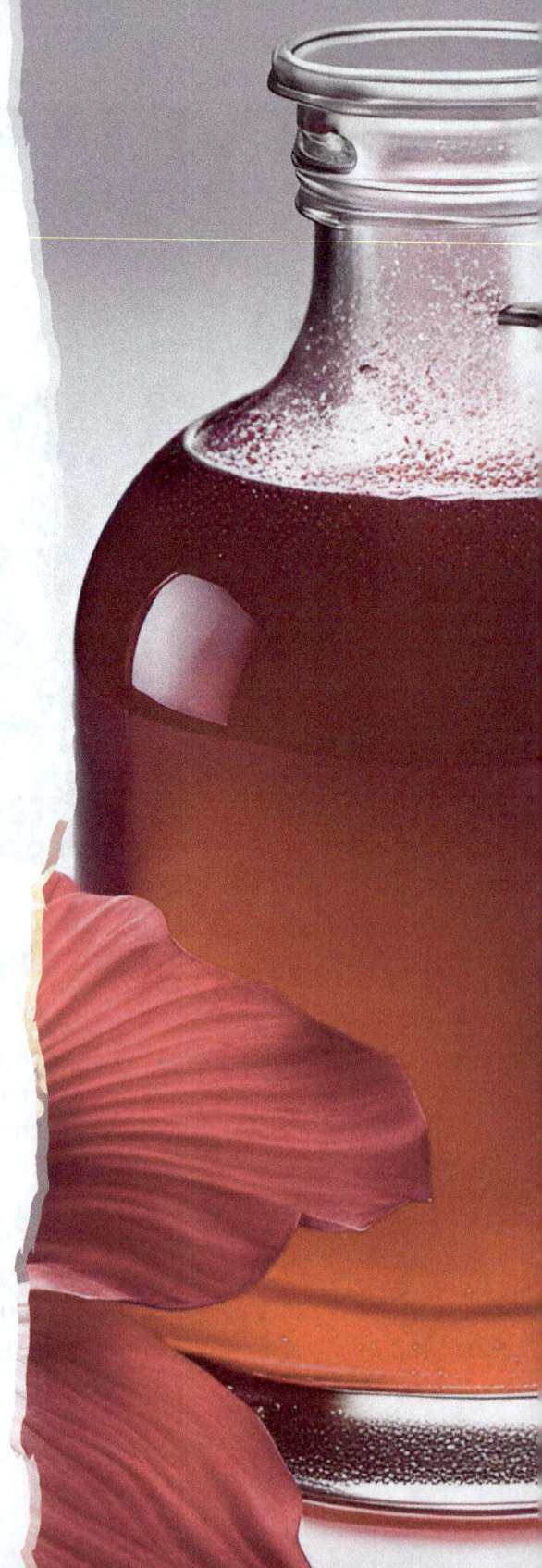

Ingredients

- 1 cup water
- 2 tablespoons dried food-grade hibiscus flowers or hibiscus tea bags

Procedure

1. Bring water to a boil, in a saucepan, then add the dried hibiscus flowers or tea bags.
2. Reduce the heat and simmer for 5 minutes. Remove from heat and let the tea steep for an additional 10 minutes.
3. Strain out the flowers and let the tea cool before pouring into a sterilized bottle or jar.
4. Store in the refrigerator.

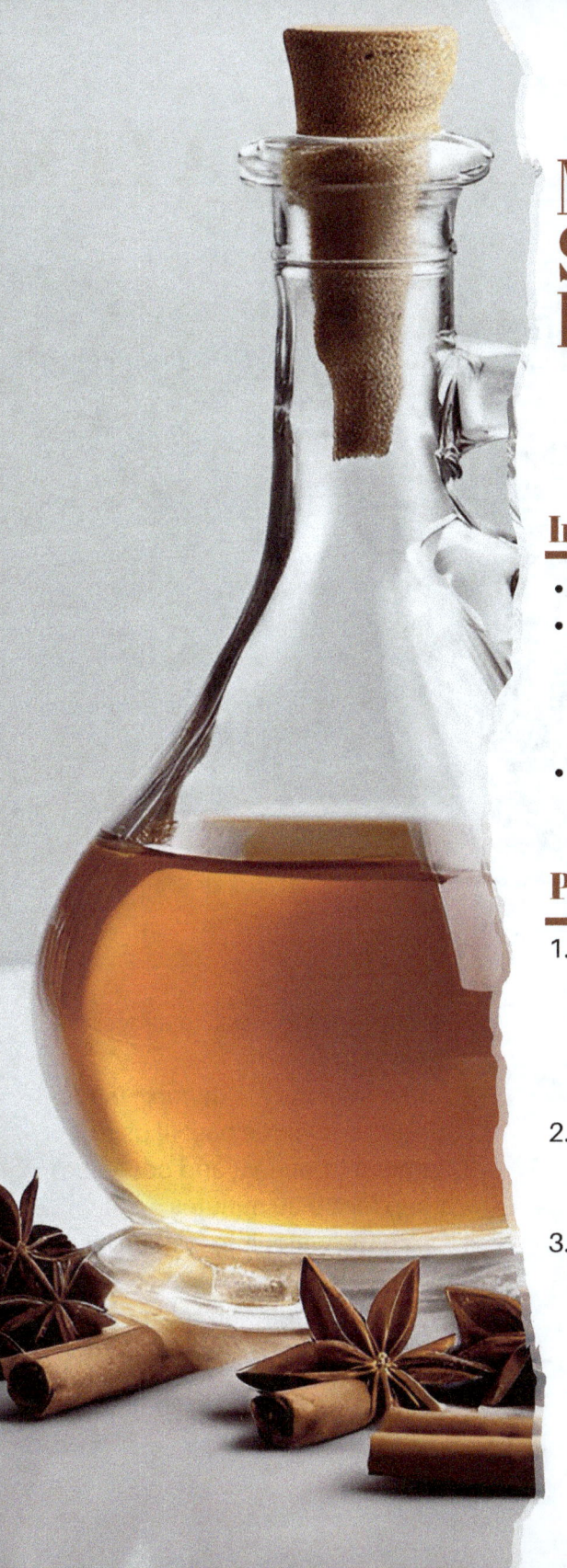

MULLING SPICE INFUSION

Ingredients

- 1 cup water
- 1 tablespoon mulling spices (cinnamon sticks, cloves, allspice berries, and star anise)
- Zest of 1 orange

Procedure

1. In a saucepan, combine water, mulling spices, and orange zest. Bring to a boil, then reduce the heat and simmer for 10 minutes.
2. Remove from heat and let the mixture steep for an additional 10 minutes.
3. Strain out the spices and pour the infusion into a sterilized bottle or jar. Store in the refrigerator for up to 2 weeks.

HERB-INFUSED WATER

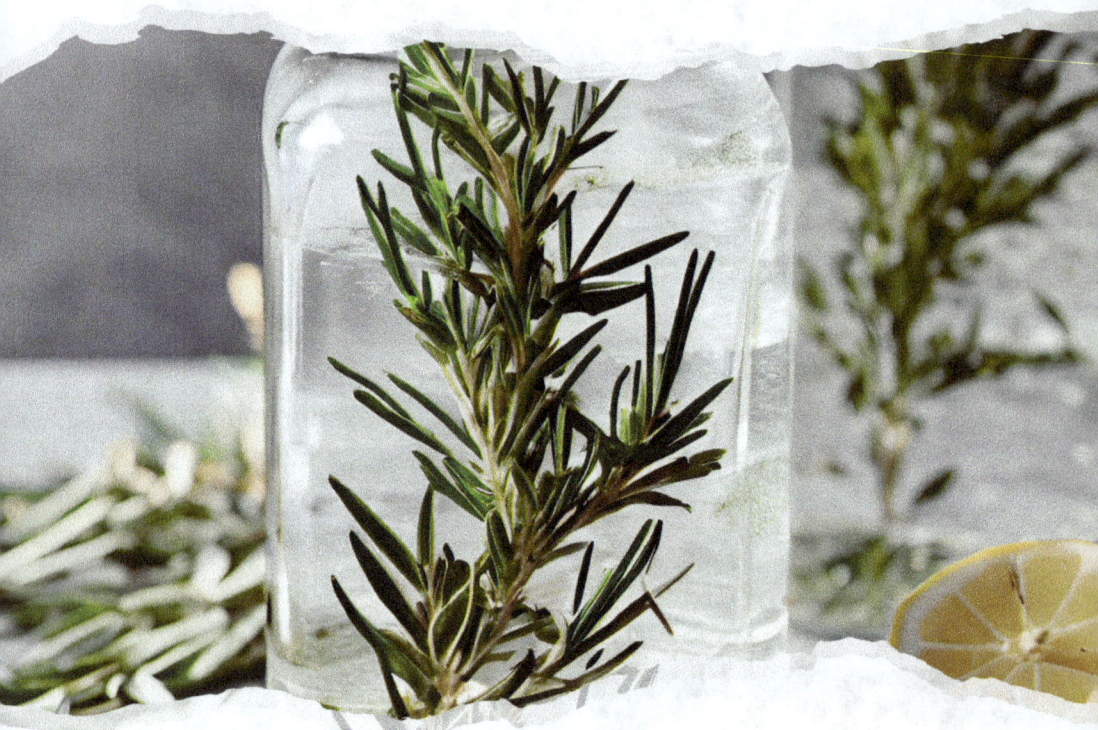

Ingredients

- 4 cups water
- 1 sprig fresh rosemary
- 1 sprig fresh thyme
- 2-3 sage leaves
- 1 small piece of ginger (optional, for a warming touch)
- 1 strip of lemon or orange peel (optional)

Procedure

1. Bring water to a boil in a medium saucepan.
2. Add rosemary, thyme, sage, ginger, and citrus peel (if using).
3. Remove from heat and cover. Let steep for 20-30 minutes.
4. Strain the water into a clean jar or pitcher and let it cool.
5. Store in the refrigerator for up to 5 days.

CHAI CONCENTRATE

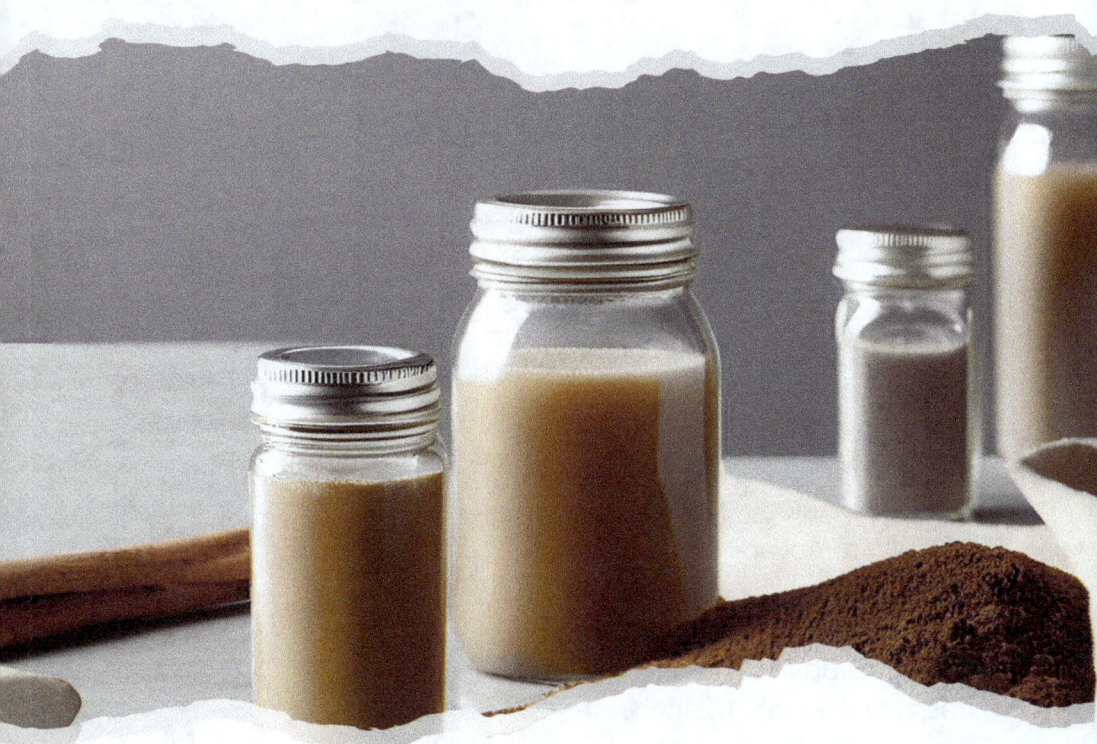

Ingredients

- 3 cups water
- 6 black tea bags (or 6 tsp loose black tea)
- 2 cinnamon sticks
- 5 whole cardamom pods, cracked
- 5 whole cloves
- 1-2 whole star anise (optional)
- 1-inch piece of fresh ginger, sliced
- 1/2 tsp black peppercorns
- 1/4 cup coconut sugar or honey (or to taste)
- 1 tsp vanilla extract

Procedure

1. In a medium saucepan, bring water to a boil.
2. Add cinnamon, cardamom, cloves, star anise, ginger, and black peppercorns.
3. Reduce heat to low, cover, and simmer for 15 minutes.
4. Add the tea bags and simmer for another 5-7 minutes.
5. Remove from heat, strain the mixture, and stir in sugar/honey and vanilla extract.
6. Store in an airtight jar in the fridge for up to 7 days.

CITRUS INFUSION

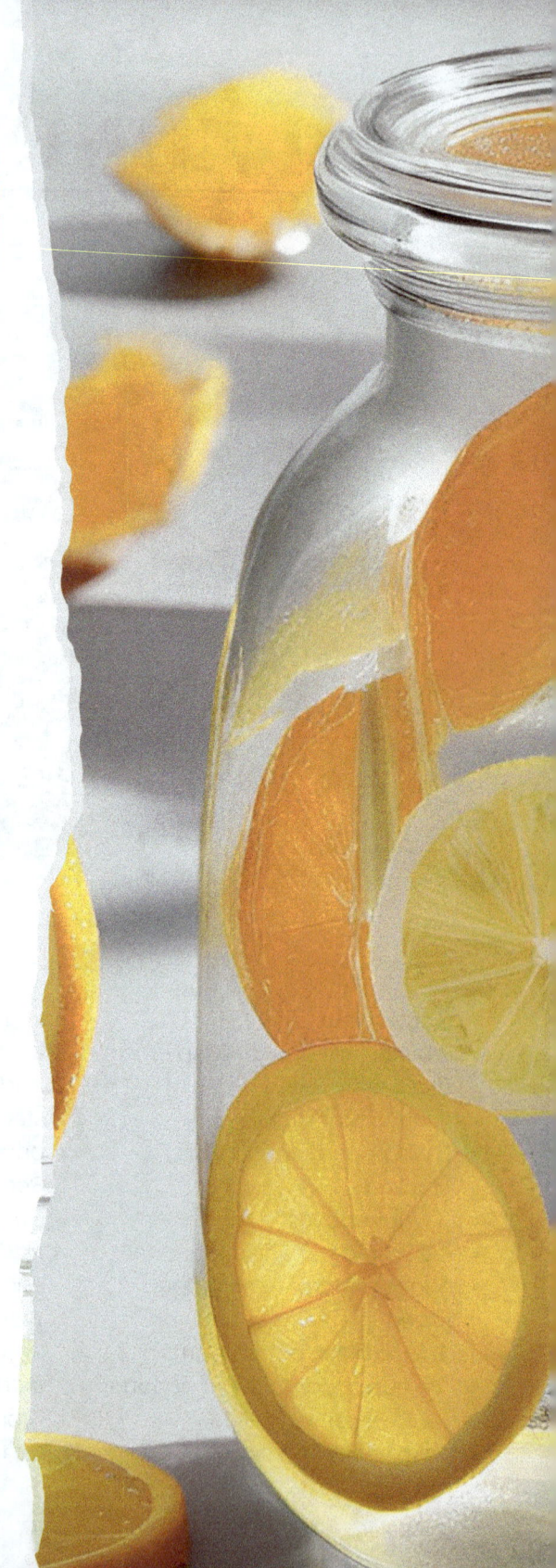

Ingredients

- 4 cups water
- 1 orange (peeled, sliced, and pith removed)
- 1 lemon (peeled, sliced, and pith removed)
- 1 lime (peeled, sliced, and pith removed)
- Optional add-ins: a few fresh mint leaves, 1/2-inch ginger, or a cinnamon stick

Procedure

1. Add all the ingredients to a medium saucepan.
2. Bring to a boil, then reduce heat to low.
3. Simmer for 10-15 minutes.
4. Remove from heat, strain, and let cool.
5. Store in a glass jar in the fridge for up to 3-5 days.

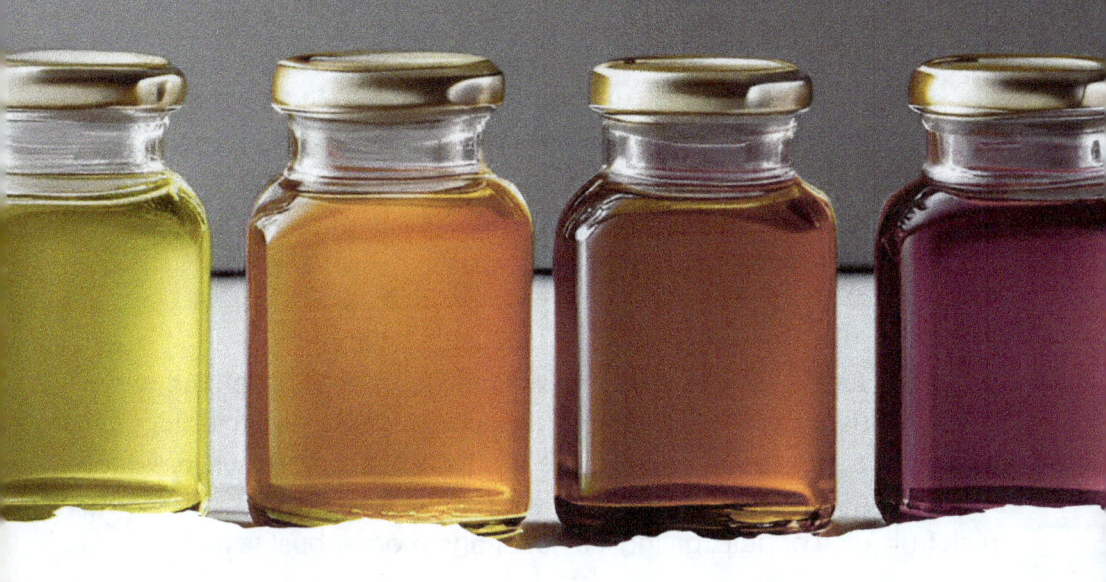

CORDIALS

Bursting with vibrant, natural flavors, these syrups capture the essence of fresh fruit, creating deliciously sweet and tangy bases for your mocktails.

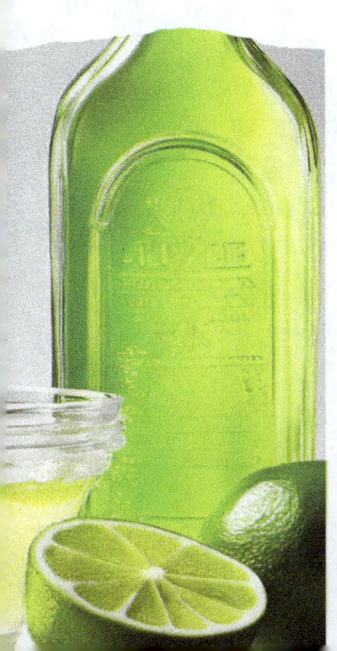
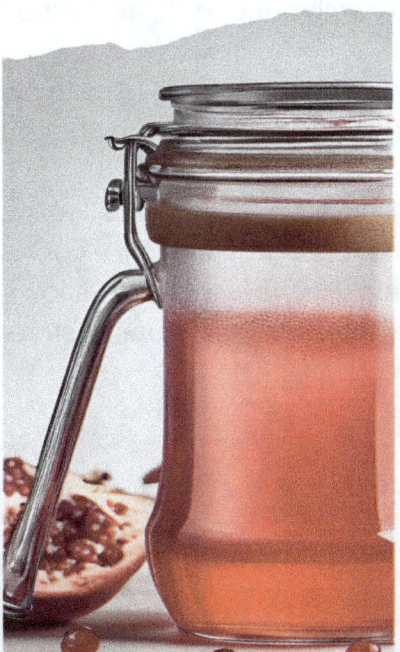
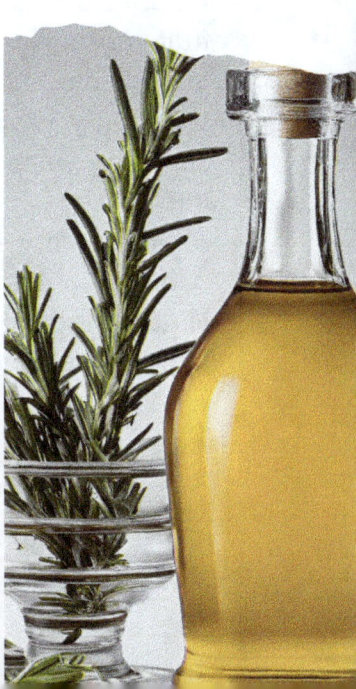

What is a Cordial?

A cordial is a concentrated, sweetened, and often fruit-based liquid that is used as a flavor enhancer in beverages and culinary applications. It is typically made by combining fruit juice, sugar, and sometimes acids (like citric acid) to create a vibrant, shelf-stable concentrate. Cordials can be used to make mocktails, cocktails, sodas, desserts, and even savory dishes.

While cordials and syrups share similarities, they are not the same. A cordial is usually more complex in flavor, sometimes including herbs, spices, or acids to enhance its depth. Unlike a simple syrup, which is primarily sugar and water infused with a flavor, a cordial often contains fresh fruit juice or pulp, giving it a richer and more robust taste.

The Purpose of Cordials in Mocktail Making

Cordials are essential building blocks in mocktail recipes because they provide depth of flavor, balance acidity and sweetness, and make it easy to create sophisticated, alcohol-free drinks.

Why Use a Cordial in a Mocktail?

- **Concentrated Flavor** – Unlike juices, which can be watery and mild, cordials are rich and intense, providing a bold flavor base or drinks.
- **Balanced Sweetness & Acidity** – Many cordials include citrus or tart fruit, ensuring a well-rounded taste without the need for extra ingredients.
- **Versatility** – A single cordial can be used in multiple ways: mixed with sparkling water for a refreshing soda, added to tea, or incorporated into desserts.
- **Shelf Stability** – Unlike fresh juice, a well-made cordial can last weeks or even months in the fridge, making it a convenient ingredient.
- **Natural Ingredient Focus** – Cordials allow you to use fresh, real ingredients rather than artificial syrups or store-bought concentrates.

Examples of Cordials in Mocktails

- Elderflower Cordial Spritz – Elderflower cordial + soda water + fresh mint
- Raspberry Lime Cooler – Raspberry cordial + fresh lime juice + tonic water
- Ginger Cordial Fizz – Ginger cordial + sparkling water + a dash of bitters

Beyond Mocktails: Other Uses for Cordials

Cordials are not just for drinks! They can enhance both sweet and savory dishes in creative ways:

In Cooking & Baking:

- Drizzle over cakes, pancakes, or ice cream for a fruit-infused touch.
- Mix into frostings, glazes, or sauces for an extra layer of flavor.
- Use in salad dressings or marinades, especially citrus or berry-based cordials.

As a DIY Soda Alternative:

- Skip artificial sodas and mix cordials with sparkling water for a natural, flavorful soda.
- Combine with herbal teas for a unique, non-alcoholic iced drink.

As a Wellness Ingredient:

- Some cordials, like ginger or elderberry, can have immune-boosting benefits when diluted in warm water or tea.
- Lemon, ginger, or honey cordials can be soothing for sore throats.

Why Every Mocktail Maker Should Have Cordials

Cordials are a powerful ingredient in mocktail crafting, offering intense flavor, balance, and versatility in a way that simple syrups or infusions cannot. Whether you're creating elegant alcohol-free drinks, refreshing sodas, or using them in the kitchen, cordials provide a natural, vibrant way to enhance flavor.

For any mocktail enthusiast, having a few homemade or high-quality store-bought cordials on hand can elevate your drink-making game and expand your creativity beyond the glass!

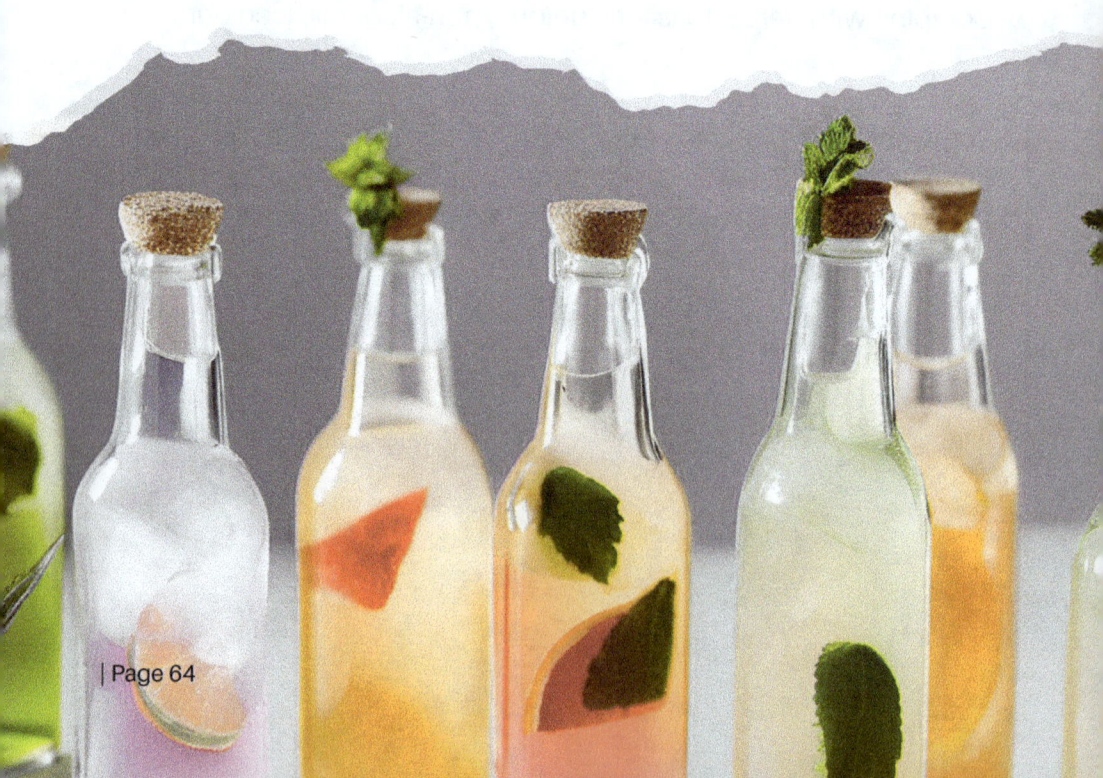

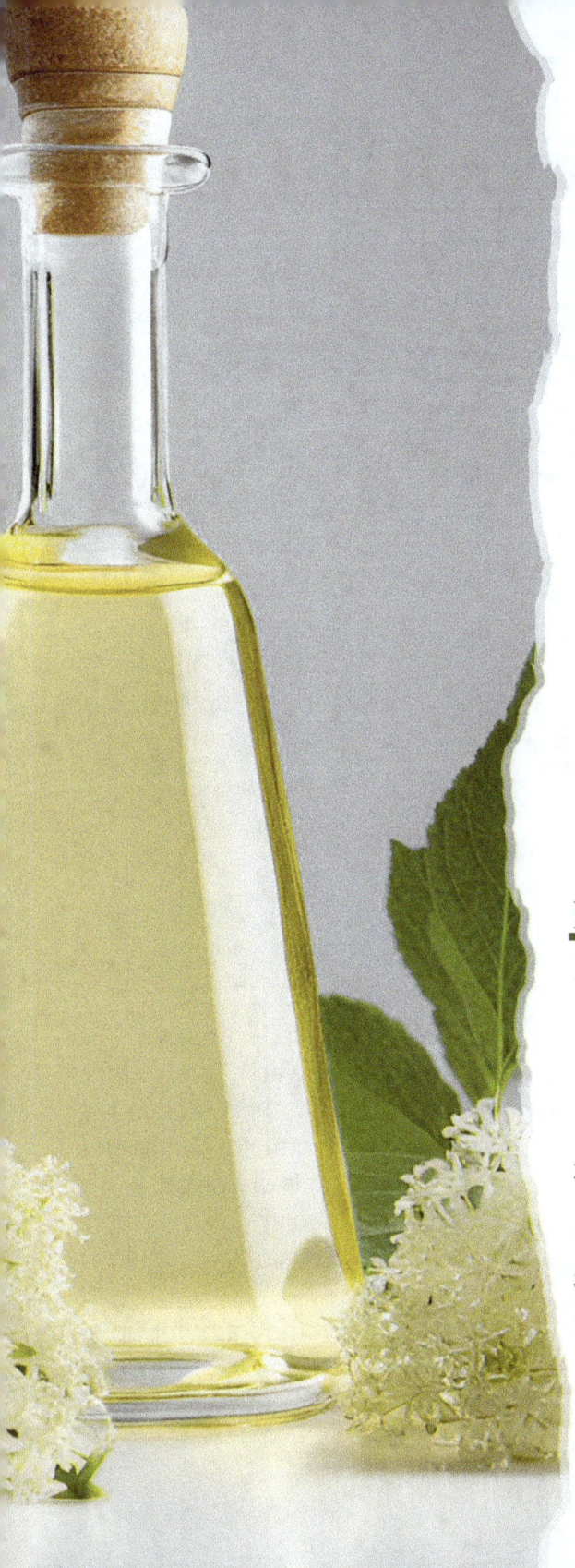

ELDER FLOWER CORDIAL

Ingredients

- 1 cup water
- 1 cup granulated sugar
- 1/2 cup dried elderflowers or 1 cup fresh elderflowers (organic and food-grade)
- Optional: Juice of 1 lemon

Procedure

1. In a saucepan, combine water, sugar, elderflowers, and lemon juice. Bring to a boil, then reduce the heat and simmer for 5 minutes.
2. Remove from heat and let the mixture steep for 15 minutes.
3. Strain out the elderflowers and let the cordial cool before pouring into a sterilized bottle or jar. Store in the refrigerator for up to 2 weeks.

LEMON CORDIAL

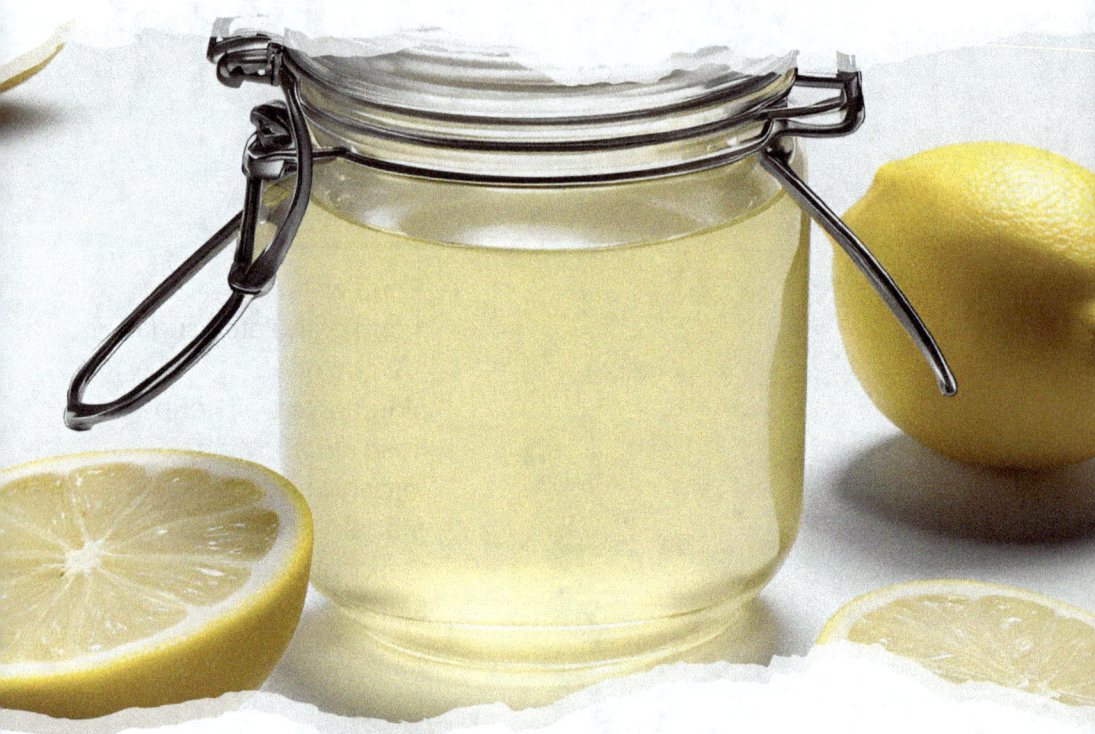

Ingredients

- 1 cup water
- 1 cup granulated sugar
- 1 cup fresh lemon juice (from about 4-5 lemons)

Procedure

1. In a saucepan, combine the lemon juice, water, and sugar. Bring to a boil, then reduce the heat and simmer for 5 minutes until the sugar is dissolved.
2. Let the cordial cool before pouring into a sterilized bottle or jar.
3. Store in the refrigerator for up to 2 weeks.

SPICED APPLE CORDIAL

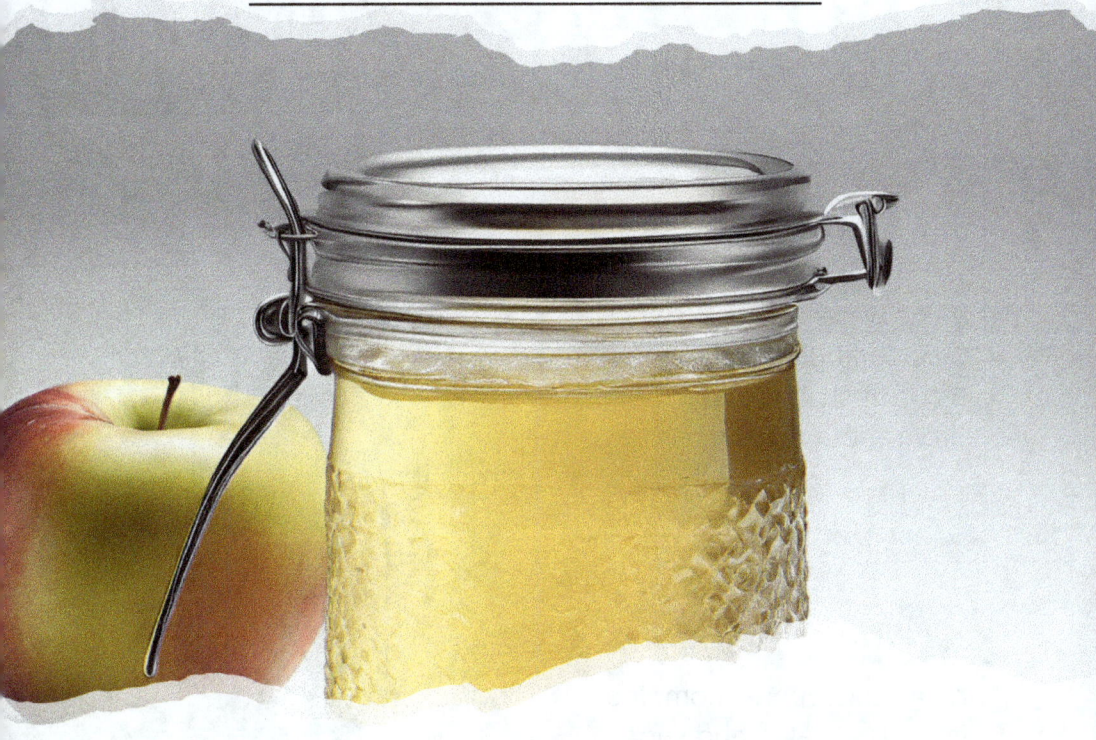

Ingredients

- 1/2 cup water
- 1/2 cup granulated sugar
- 1 cup fresh apple juice
- 1 cinnamon stick
- 3 whole cloves
- 1 star anise

Procedure

1. In a saucepan, combine apple juice, water, sugar, and spices.
2. Bring the mixture to a boil, then reduce the heat and simmer for 10 minutes.
3. Remove from heat and let the cordial steep for 15 minutes.
4. Strain out the spices and pour the cordial into a sterilized bottle or jar.
5. Store in the refrigerator for up to 1 week.

LIME CORDIAL

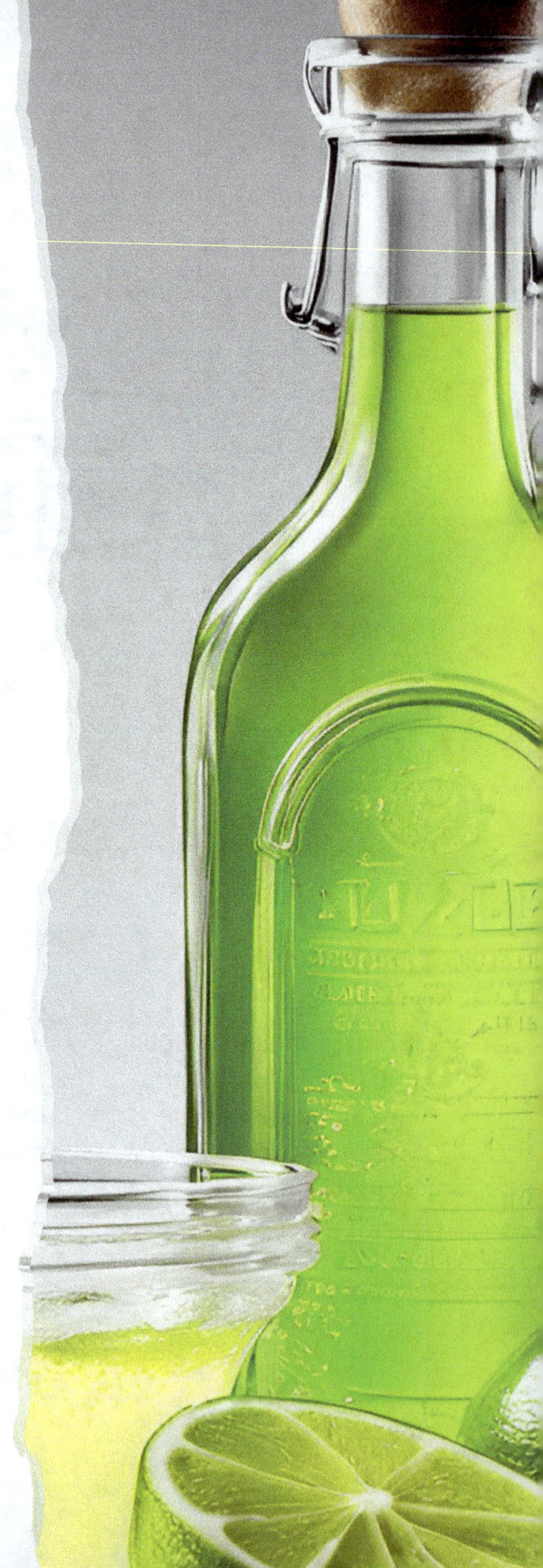

Ingredients

- 1 cup water
- 1 cup granulated sugar
- 1 cup fresh lime juice (from about 8-10 limes)

Procedure

1. In a saucepan, combine lime juice, water, and sugar. Bring to a boil, then reduce the heat and simmer for 5 minutes until the sugar is dissolved.
2. Let the cordial cool before pouring into a sterilized bottle or jar.
3. Store in the refrigerator for up to 2 weeks.

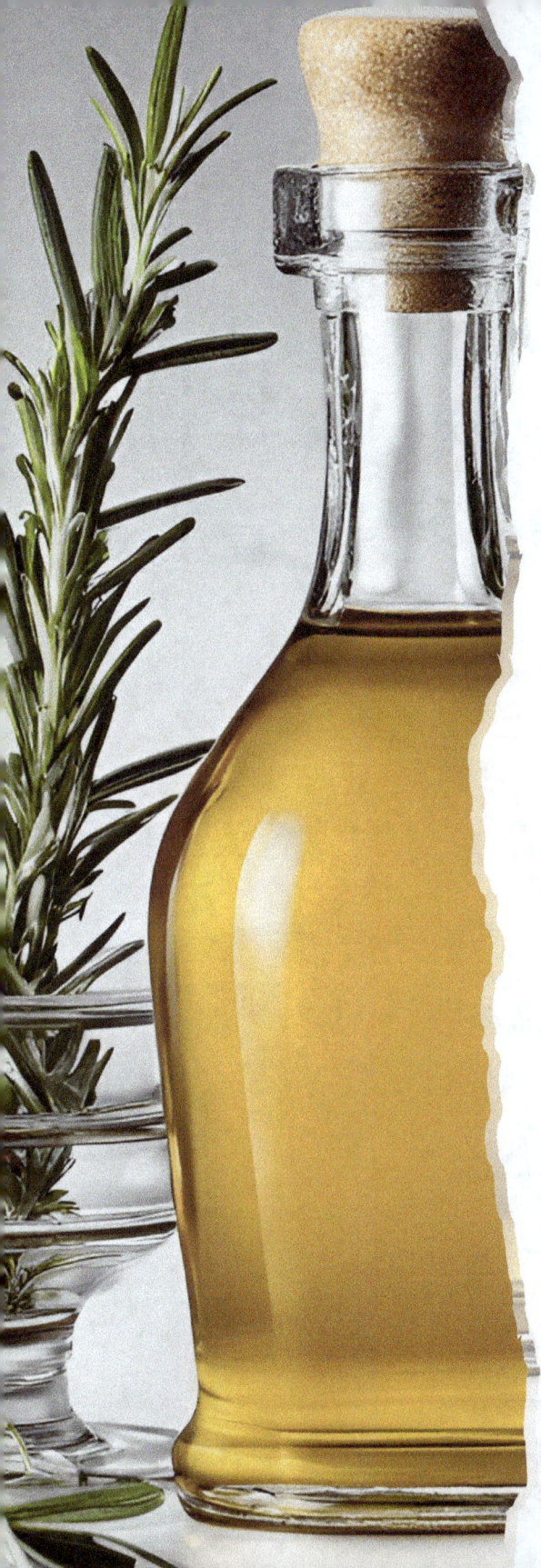

ROSEMARY CORDIAL

Ingredients

- 1 cup water
- 1 cup granulated sugar
- 3 sprigs fresh rosemary
- Optional: Zest of 1 orange or lemon, as preferred.

Procedure

1. In a saucepan, combine the water, sugar, rosemary sprigs, and orange/lemon zest (if using).
2. Bring the mixture to a boil, then reduce the heat and simmer for 5 minutes.
3. Remove from heat and let it steep for 15 minutes.
4. Strain out the rosemary and zest, then pour the cordial into a sterilized bottle or jar.
5. Store in the refrigerator for up to 2 weeks.

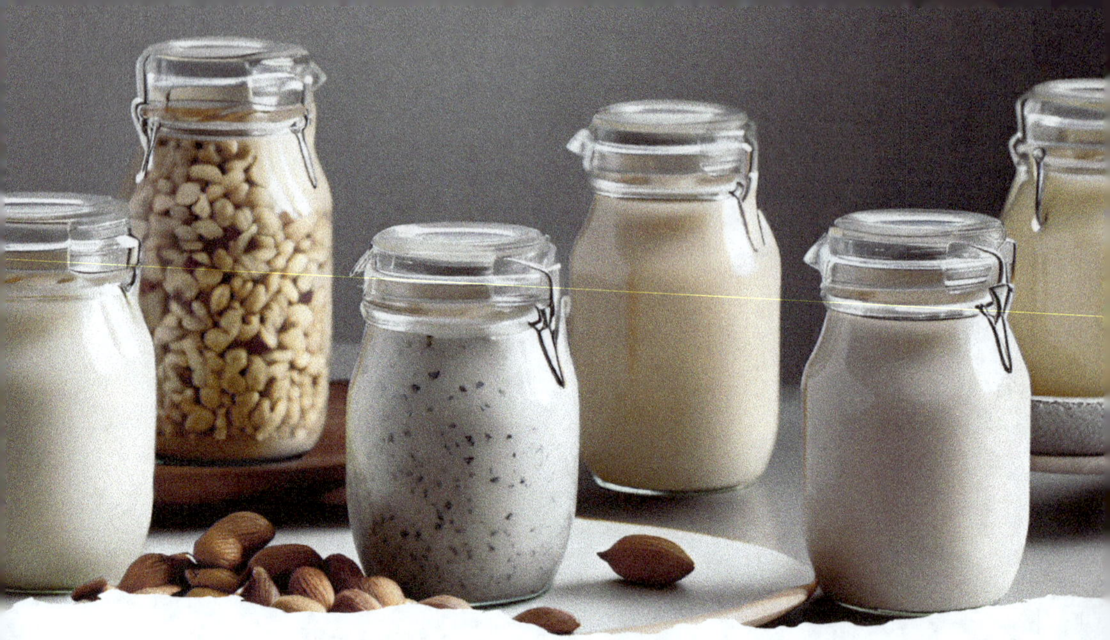

NUT MILKS

Rich, creamy, and naturally delicious, these dairy-free alternatives add smoothness and body to mocktails, hot drinks, and indulgent seasonal sips.

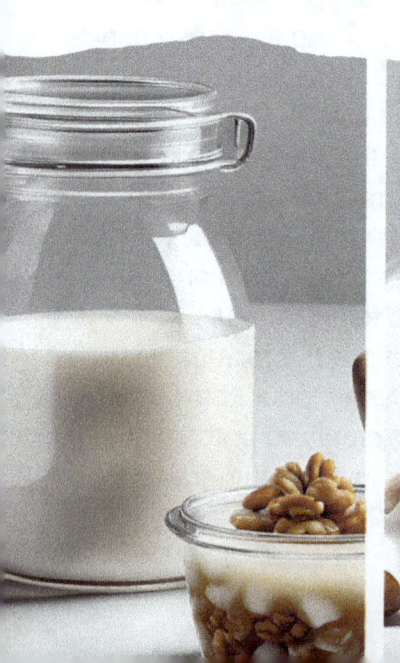
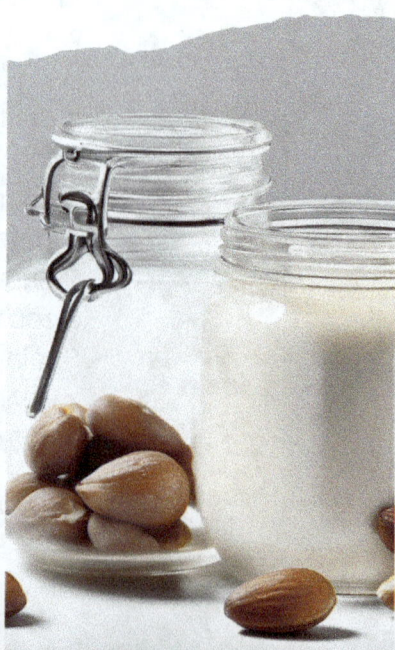
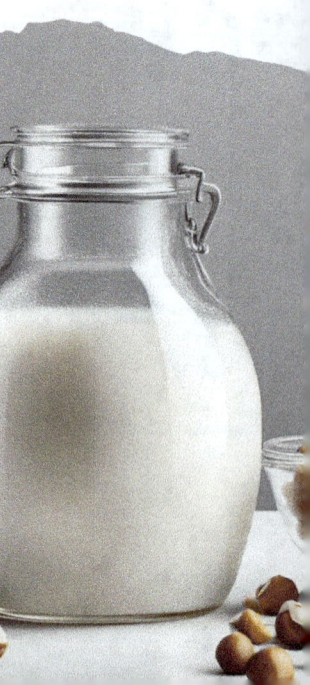

What are nut milks?

Homemade nut milks are non-dairy, fresh, flavorful, and generally free from preservatives. Each recipe can be sweetened or otherwise flavored to suit your taste.

Experiment with a few and enjoy these rich, smooth, buttery and creamy flavorful additions to your Mocktails and more!

Typical uses for nut milks are in smoothies, lattes, hot chocolate, oatmeal or cereals, soups, sauces, baking, or they can be quite delicious on their own.

- **Shelf Life:** All of these nut milks last 3-4 days in the fridge if stored in a sterilized, airtight glass jar.
- **Separation:** Nut milk naturally separates, so just give it a shake before use.
- **Freezing:** You can freeze nut milk in ice cube trays for use in smoothies later.

When we think of mocktails, our minds often go straight to fruity, bubbly, or citrus-based drinks. But with nut milks, there's an entirely different world of rich, creamy, and luxurious mocktails! Using nut milks in mocktails allows you to create indulgent, dessert-like flavors.

These plant-based milks add a silky texture, natural sweetness, and a depth of flavor that elevate your alcohol-free drinks to something truly special.

Why Use Nut Milks in Mocktails?

Nut milks milk offer a creamy, velvety texture that blends beautifully into both hot and cold mocktails. They work particularly well in:

- **Velvety dessert mocktails:** Think vanilla, cinnamon, or chocolate-based drinks.
- **Tropical blends:** Coconut or almond milk adds richness to fruity mocktails.
- **Spiced warm drinks:** Perfect for chai, golden turmeric lattes, or Mexican hot chocolate mocktails.
- **Smooth, balanced creations:** Nut milk is naturally sweet and helps tone down acidic or bitter flavors.

Additionally, nut milks are dairy-free, making them a fantastic alternative for anyone who is lactose-intolerant or prefers plant-based options. If you prefer to use dairy, you can just substitute it in.

Some Types of Nut Milks for Mocktails

- **Coconut Milk:** Rich and tropical, coconut milk pairs well with pineapple, mango, vanilla, lime, and rum-style flavors. A splash of coconut milk can make a mocktail feel like a creamy piña colada without the alcohol.
- **Almond Milk:** Lightly nutty and slightly sweet, almond milk is incredibly versatile. It complements vanilla, caramel, cinnamon, berries, and even citrus when balanced correctly.
- **Cashew Milk:** Ultra-creamy and naturally buttery, cashew milk adds depth and smoothness to mocktails. It works beautifully in coffee-based, chocolate, or nut-flavored drinks.
- **Hazelnut Milk:** A rich and fragrant choice, hazelnut milk enhances mocha-style mocktails, chocolate blends, and even spiced drinks.

How to Use Nut & Milks in Mocktails
- **Shaken & Blended:** Add nut or oamilk to a cocktail shaker with ice and shake for a smooth, frothy texture.
- **Steamed & Frothed:** Use a frother to create a silky foam for hot mocktails like chai lattes or golden milk.
- **Layered:** Gently pour over fruit purées or coffee for a beautiful, layered effect.
- **Frozen:** Blend with frozen fruit and ice for a creamy, slushy-style drink.

Flavor Pairings & Inspiration
- **Fresh & Herbal:** Almond or cashew milk + lavender, vanilla, or rose syrup.
- **Rich & Spiced:** Hazelnut milk + cinnamon, nutmeg, or cardamom.
- **Tropical & Refreshing:** Coconut milk + pineapple, mango, or passionfruit.
- **Decadent & Dessert-Like:** Cashew or hazelnut milk + chocolate, caramel, or espresso.

Mocktail Ideas Using Nut Milks
- **Golden Turmeric Latte Mocktail:** Any nut milk, turmeric, cinnamon, ginger, honey.
- **Coconut Chai Cooler:** Coconut milk, chai spice syrup, vanilla, and crushed ice.
- **Hazelnut Mocha Mocktail:** Hazelnut milk, cocoa, cold brew coffee, maple syrup.
- **Berry Almond Dream:** Almond milk, muddled berries, vanilla syrup, lemon zest.

Whether you're craving something light and refreshing or rich and indulgent, nut milks add versatility and creaminess to your mocktails. Experiment with different flavors, textures, and techniques to create one-of-a-kind alcohol-free drinks that feel as luxurious as any cocktail!

MACADAMIA NUT MILK

Ingredients

- 1 cup raw macadamia nuts (soaked for 4-8 hours)
- 4 cups filtered water
- Pinch of salt
- Optional: 1-2 dates
- Optional: 1/2 tsp vanilla extract

Procedure

1. Soak macadamia nuts for 4-8 hours.
2. Drain and rinse.
3. Blend with 4 cups of fresh water, salt, plus dates, and vanilla if using, for 1-2 minutes.
4. Strain using a nut milk bag or fine mesh sieve.
5. Store in a sterilized glass bottle in the fridge for up to 4 days.

CLASSIC ALMOND MILK

Ingredients

- 1 cup raw almonds (soaked overnight)
- 4 cups filtered water
- 1-2 dates (optional for sweetness)
- 1/2 tsp vanilla extract (optional)
- Pinch of salt

Procedure

1. Soak almonds in water overnight (or for at least 8 hours).
2. Drain and rinse the almonds.
3. Blend almonds with 4 cups of fresh filtered water, dates, vanilla, and salt for 1-2 minutes.
4. Strain using a nut milk bag, cheesecloth, or fine mesh sieve.
5. Store in a glass bottle in the fridge for up to 4 days.

BRAZIL NUT MILK

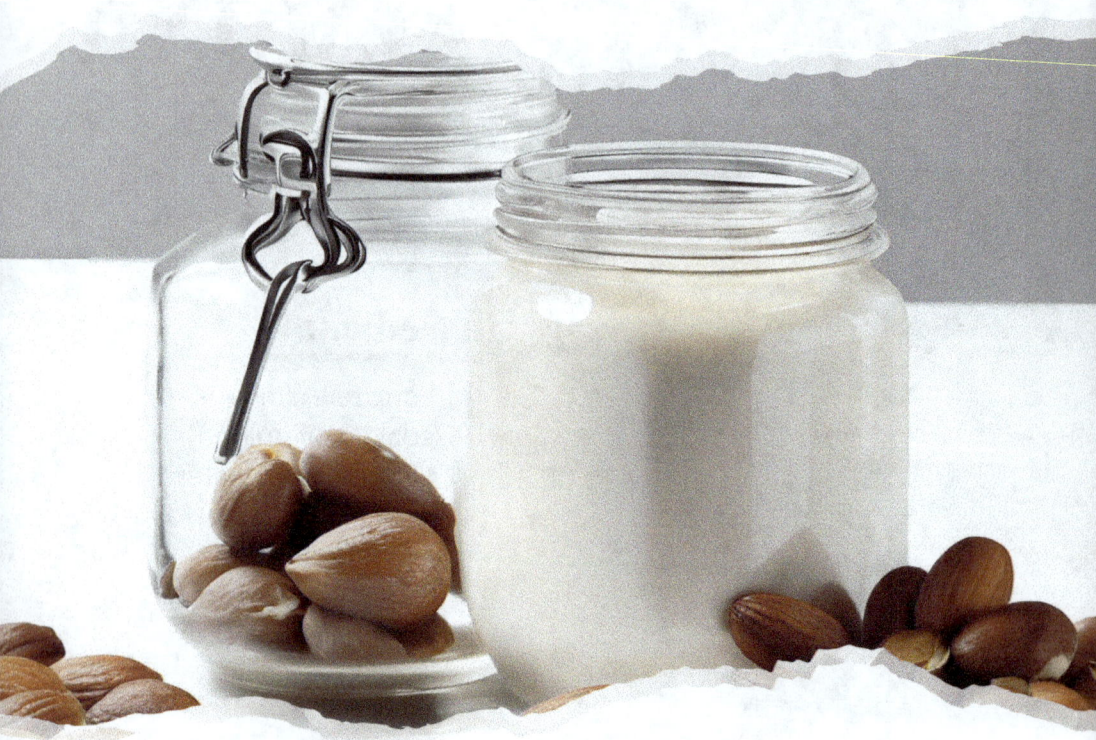

Ingredients

- 1 cup raw brazil nuts (soaked for 4-8 hours)
- 4 cups filtered water
- Pinch of salt
- Optional: 1 tsp vanilla extract
- Optional: 1 tbsp honey or maple syrup

Procedure

1. Soak brazil nuts for 4-8 hours.
2. Drain and rinse.
3. Blend nuts with 4 cups of fresh water, salt, plus sweetener and vanilla, if using, for 1-2 minutes.
4. Strain using a nut milk bag or fine mesh sieve.
5. Store in a sterilized glass bottle in the fridge for up to 4 days.

TOASTED HAZELNUT MILK

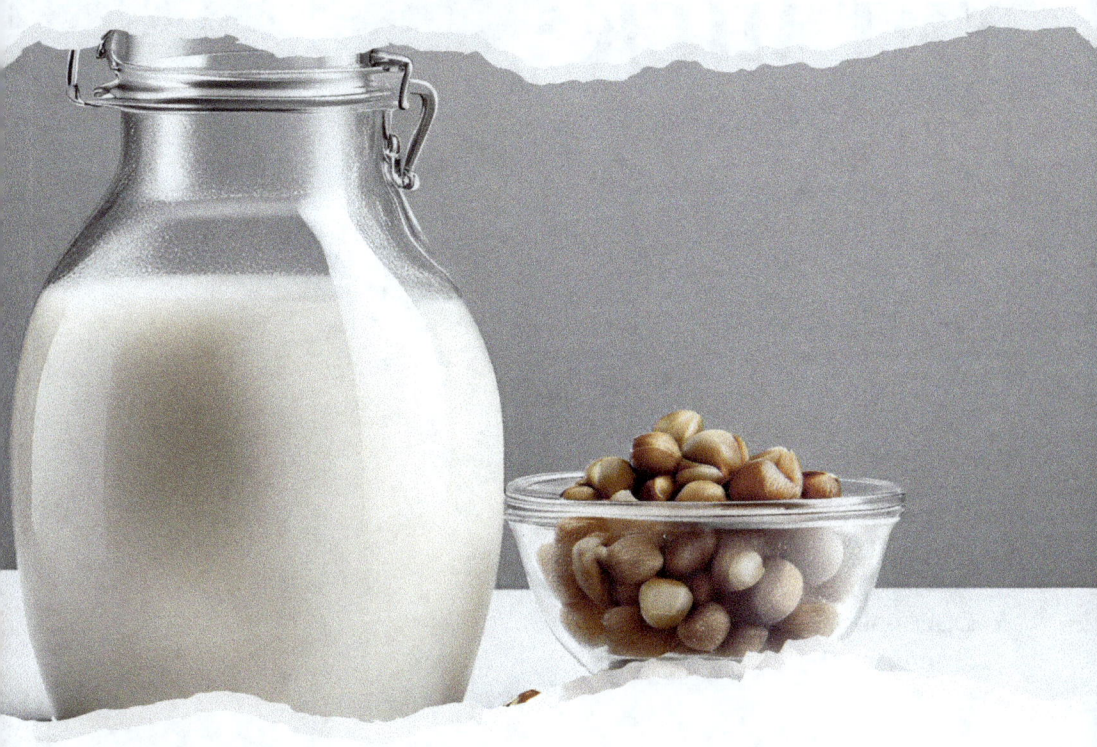

Ingredients

- 1 cup raw hazelnuts (toasted for deeper flavor)
- 4 cups filtered water
- Pinch of salt
- Optional: 1/2 tsp vanilla extract
- Optional: 1 tbsp maple syrup

Procedure

1. Toast hazelnuts in a dry pan for 5-7 minutes (optional for more flavor).
2. Soak hazelnuts for 8 hours or overnight.
3. Drain and rinse.
4. Blend with 4 cups of fresh water, maple syrup, salt, plus syrup and vanilla if using, for 1-2 minutes.
5. Strain using a nut milk bag or fine sieve.
6. Store in a sterilized glass bottle in the fridge for up to 4 days.

PECAN NUT MILK

Ingredients

- 1 cup raw pecans (soaked for 4-6 hours)
- 4 cups filtered water
- Pinch of salt
- Optional: 1 tbsp maple syrup
- Optional: 1/2 tsp ground cinnamon

Procedure

1. Toast the pecans in a dry skillet over medium heat for 3-5 minutes, until fragrant.
2. Blend the toasted pecans with water plus syrup and cinnamon if used, in a high-speed blender until smooth.
3. Strain the mixture through a nut milk bag or fine mesh sieve. Store in a sterilized glass bottle in the refrigerator for up to 3 days.

WALNUT MILK

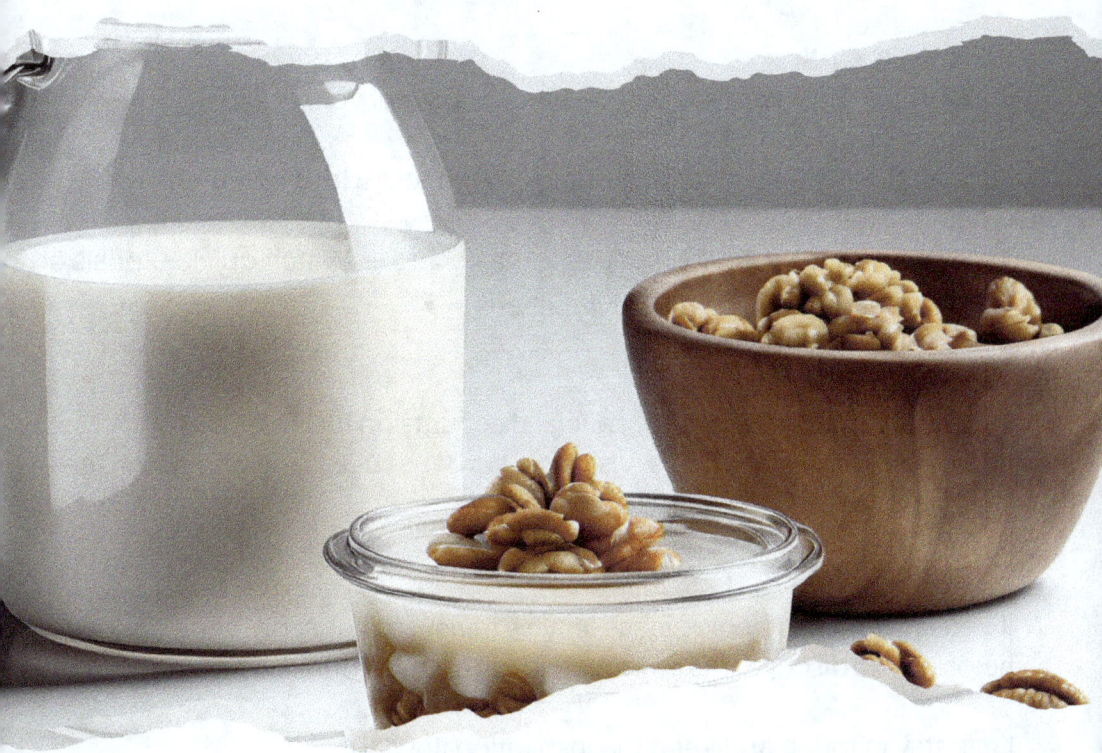

Ingredients

- 1 cup raw walnuts (soaked for 6-8 hours)
- 4 cups filtered water
- Pinch of salt
- Optional: 1-2 dates
- Optional: 1/2 tsp vanilla extract

Procedure

1. Soak walnuts for 6-8 hours.
2. Drain and rinse.
3. Blend with 4 cups of fresh water, salt, plus dates, vanilla, if using, for 1-2 minutes.
4. Strain using a nut milk bag or fine mesh sieve.
5. Store in a sterilized glass bottle in the fridge for up to 4 days.

How to Stay Connected

Love our *Syrups & Cordials*? Stay connected for updates, new recipes, and exclusive content.

Follow Us Online

Instagram : @greensaucepub — Share photos of your creations with Syrups & Cordials

Facebook : @greensaucepublishing — Connect with a community of other mcoktail drink lovers.

TikTok and Youtube : @greensaucepublishing — Watch quick tutorials on how to prepare your favorite mocktails drinks.

Join Our Newsletter

Sign up for exclusive recipes, special discounts on future books, and behind-the- scenes updates. Visit **www.greensaucepublishing.com** to sign up.

Leave a Review

If you enjoyed this book, please leave a review on Amazon. Your feedback helps others discover the warmth and joy of these drinks.

Let's stay in touch and keep the inspiration flowing!

Cheers to your mocktail adventures,

The Green Sauce Publishing Team

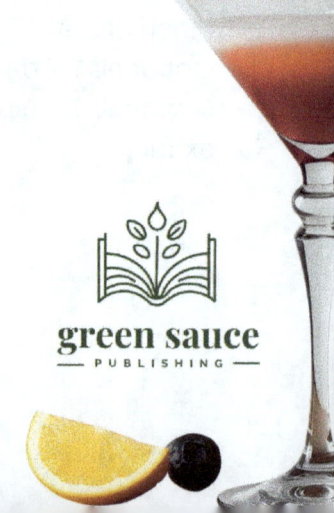

ALSO AVAILABLE

Syrups & Cordials for Mocktails is the third book in our Mocktails for Every Day Series. Check out the other books in the series, already published, or coming soon, by scanning the QR Code on page 80!

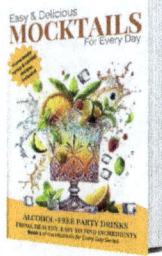

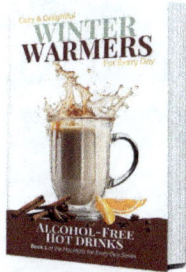

Easy & Delicious Mocktails for Every Day

Explore a world of vibrant, alcohol-free cocktails that prove fun and sophistication don't require spirits. Using fresh, easy-to-find ingredients, you'll craft party-ready drinks, from fruity infusions to zesty syrups.

Cozy & Delightful Winter Warmers

Warm and Cozy, comforting and delicious. Our Winter Warmers are just perfect for long Winter evenings or cozy Winter mornings, or any occasion with friends and family.

COMING SOON

The Mocktails for Every Day Series is growing! Use the QR Code on page 80 to sign up for notifications so you can be the first to know when the new books are published.

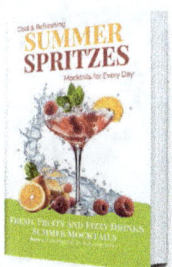

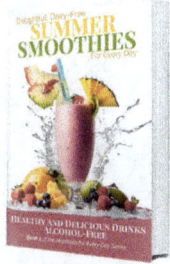

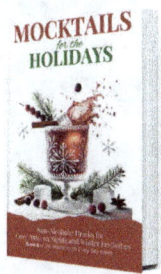

Cool & Refreshing Summer Spritzes Mocktails for Every Day

Thirst quenching, beautiful and delicious. Our Summer Spritzes are the perfect alcohol-free accompaniment for any occasion, for anyone.

Delightful Dairy-Free Summer Smoothies

Deliciously creamy, but 100% Dairy Free, our Delicious Dairy-Free Summer Smoothies will take your summer mornings to the next level!

Mocktails for the Holidays

The ultimate Holiday Mocktail recipe book for any holiday occasion, or just for a fun and festive party for one. A perfect holiday gift too!

www.ingramcontent.com/pod-product-compliance
Lightning Source LLC
LaVergne TN
LVHW022325080426
835508LV00013BA/1326